BACK IN ACTION
SARAH KEY

Back in Action

SARAH KEY

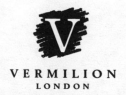

VERMILION
LONDON

1 3 5 7 9 10 8 6 4 2

Copyright © Field Mill Holdings Ltd 1986, 1990, 1991

First published in Australia and New Zealand in 1986 by Bantam Press
First published in the United Kingdom in 2001 by Vermilion
an imprint of Ebury Press
The Random House Group Ltd.
Random House, 20 Vauxhall Bridge Road, London SW1V 2SA

Random House Australia (Pty) Limited
20 Alfred Street, Milsons Point, Sydney,
New South Wales 2061, Australia

Random House New Zealand Limited
18 Poland Road, Glenfield,
Auckland 10, New Zealand

Random House (Pty) Limited
Endulini, 5A Jubilee Road, Parktown 2193, South Africa

The Random House Group Limited Reg. No. 954009
www.randomhouse.co.uk

A CIP catalogue record for this book is available from the British Library.

ISBN: 0 09 185997 2

Typeset by SX Composing DTP, Rayleigh, Essex
Printed and bound in Great Britain by Mackays of Chatham Plc, Chatham, Kent

Papers used by Vermilion are natural, recyclable products
made from wood grown in sustainable forests.

To my four children;
Jemima, Harry, Freddie
and Scarlett

Disclaimer

Anyone who feels excessive strain or pain on attempting any of the exercises described in this book or who is under medical supervision for back trouble is recommended only to follow the exercises subject to the approval of their doctor.

Foreword

ST. JAMES'S PALACE

British industry is said to lose more man-hours of otherwise productive time through 'bad backs' than through any other cause, yet I am told that the understanding of human back disorders has hardly advanced at all in the last 30 years. So it is encouraging to encounter the refreshingly direct approach which Sarah Key, as a physiotherapist, adopts in this interesting and challenging book. Speaking directly to the sufferers, and there must be literally millions of us who do suffer from time to time in this way, she explains the problems using easy-to-understand layman's terms.

Of course, there will always be people who disapprove when collective conventional thinking is challenged, in the field of medicine or any other area for that matter, but there must surely be a place for common sense and a 'natural' non-invasive approach, based on an intimate knowledge of the musculo-skeletal system, alongside the more conventional treatments. This book certainly suggests that there is, as do many people who have been helped by the techniques of manipulation which it advocates. At this point I must stress that I am writing as someone whose back has been infinitely improved by Sarah Key's ministrations, not to mention my arm . . .! However, the treatment also involves a great deal of hard work and application on the part of the patient!

Acknowledgements

When previous editions of *Back in Action* were completed and in the bookshops, I began to lament my lack of acknowledgement of the people past and present who helped me turn my youthful fascination with backs into a consuming interest, indeed a whole way of life. With that in mind, and the opportunity offered by recent editions, I would like to express my thanks to some special individuals.

There were some who, it could be said, gave this young hitch hiker lifts along the way: Alec Sinclair, the New Zealand doctor at King's College Hospital in London, who taught me the first essentials of spinal manipulation; Greg Grieve who, with his mellifluous delivery, brought language and lyricism to the dessicated world of orthopaedic medicine; Geoff Maitland, the Australian pioneer and 'Prophet . . . save in his own land', who put manual therapy on the map; and, finally, the academics Lance Twomey and Nikolai Bogduk, two brilliant men who have brought critical analysis to the fore, helping to back up an art with science without necessarily turning it into one. And then there are the patients - not just bodies but real men and women who put their faith and trust in me. They're the ones who really taught me. I hope you find this edition even more informative than previous ones.

Sarah Key
April 2000

Contents

Introduction

HOW THIS BOOK CAME ABOUT

In March 1973 I left my native Sydney to go 'overseas'. There is nothing unusual in that; lots of young Australians do it. At the airport I cried buckets of tears, but I knew I had to go. I had something to do and I knew I had to leave to do it. Sometimes you have to leave to set free a murmur inside. That very murmur might instantly be swept away, lost in a chilling eddy of thin foreign air, but at least it had a chance, away from the close scrutiny of 'home'. Sometimes it is easier to make a go of things on someone else's pitch. I was going to London.

I made my journey to England overland across Africa. We were travelling in long-wheelbase Land Rovers and making a very slow job of it. We were inching across the northern part of Zaire when, one evening as the heat was fading from the day, I sat idly watching as one of our party fell asleep upright in her seat. Her head lolled heavily to one side as the vehicle lurched clumsily over red earth roads which were narrow and deeply pot-holed and overhung with a dense tangle of jungle greenery. We camped that evening, and the night passed, but the next day she woke barely able to move her neck. Because I was a physiotherapist, the group looked to me to 'do something' and, frankly, I could do nothing. Beyond offering vague forms of massage and a few words of solace, I was as much help as anyone else in the group. I felt useless. Like so many people who spend their life grappling with a spinal problem I, too, was in the dark, lost in the wilderness, not knowing what to do for the best.

But a clear distillate of purpose pooled in my mind. I realised then with absolute clarity what I must do in life. In that stiff spine, something stiffened in me – the resolve to quietly pursue a single goal. I was not ambitious; I just never changed my mind. My mission was to find out a thing or two about human spines – those elegant, delicately poised mechanisms that so often go wrong. Why did they go wrong? And were there not simple measures to follow when they went off the rails? Or would there always be only two options: either doing nothing or doing something drastic? Surely there must be some wide, welcoming, middle road out there for the taking.

Looking back, I often think that my personal road to Damascus was deep in the heart of the African jungle. The longer we dallied there, the keener I became. I flew into London from Tunis to be greeted by the 1973 heatwave. It was quite unlike the London I came to know. Everyone was hurrying about with great hope and cheer, as people do in the Northern Hemisphere with the smile of unaccustomed sun on their backs.

It was the end of July and it was hot. In the Tube during the rush hour, it was every bit as sticky as the Central African Republic had been two months before. But I remember being exhilarated with my new-found purpose in life. This exciting city, with its red double-decker buses and 'Monopoly' names like Pall Mall and Park Lane, was to be my home for many years. It was the maze I was to wander through in my search for knowledge. It was exhilarating, all right!

I was as poor as a church mouse. I lived with a motley collection of itinerant Australians in a cold and echoing house in Kilburn, north London. What a mixed bag we were. One was a barmaid, another a builder's labourer, another a reporter/photographer for *The Australian* newspaper in London. Others worked in Harrods selling stockings. Just about everybody earned more than me; physiotherapy was a poorly rated trade.

I went for various job interviews; there were many hospitals crying out for staff, but I only wanted to go where I could glean some knowledge. I had heard that the Royal National Orthopaedic Hospital in Great Portland Street was the place to be but there were no vacancies at the time and I did not get to work there until two years later.

Meanwhile I fell sick with infectious hepatitis, a legacy of my trip through Africa. For three weeks I was barricaded into a single room in the Middlesex Hospital in Mortimer Street and barrier-nursed. My only company all day was a book called *Vertebral Manipulation* by G. D. Maitland, and I read it from cover to cover, inside out, throughout that lonely time.

That book supercharged me with adrenalin; I could hardly wait to get out there among the groaning mass of back sufferers because, according to this book, it all seemed so logical. It was all in the hands!

I didn't care where I worked, just as long as I worked, and Outpatients was the best, with patients obligingly offering up their spines for me to have a go on. My first job was at the St Leonards Hospital in the East End of London. It was probably one of the most run-down and neglected hospitals in the land. I remember you walked straight off the street into a vast staff dining room with walls lined floor to ceiling with shiny pale blue tiles, so that it resembled a huge fish-tank. A few sleepy hospital porters sat reading newspapers and muttering to one another in monotones, and nobody could direct me to Physiotherapy. However, I was as happy as a sandboy to be working there. Long-suffering patients who had previously been turned away with a sad shake of the head, or, worse still, ineffectively treated with heat and light, doggedly re-presented themselves in the hope that modern medicine had finally conjured up something new – even if that something was me, tentatively feeling my way around with the book open at the right page.

In 1976, I opened the doors of my own private consulting rooms in Weymouth Street, in the Harley Street area of London. They were two rooms on the second floor, accessed via a cranky old lift with a concertina wire-grille door. The rooms themselves were completely bare but pleasant and airy. The contents were one desk, two chairs and a treatment couch. These and a pair of hands – the simple tools of the trade.

The way seemed clear ahead. I had nothing to lose. I still had no money but I had lots of time to tinker. I calculated that I only needed to see a few patients a day to pay the rent, with some left over to live on, so things could only get better. Besides, it was far better to be seeing the increasing numbers of patients referred by consultants from the Orthopaedic Hospital at a proper professional address, rather than at their homes or in hotel rooms.

And the English are pretty partial to us Aussies. They smile on us in mild amusement, rather like an indulgent benefactor observing an unruly child, and it seemed easy to make a go of things. Two and a half decades later, I no longer have my clinic in the heart of Harley Street with cars double and treble parked outside. Instead, I spend hours on jet planes, seeing people in far off lands and talking to patients and practitioners alike through my website in Sydney.

I have learnt there is no shortage of back sufferering. I have also learnt that most backs can be diagnosed and treated using the hands. Yes, the hands – that most ancient form of healing, so long relegated to a therapeutic backwater. I have learnt there is hope for the people who were previously sent off with pills, or dispatched with feeble exercises in the hope of loosening things up (only to find when the enthusiasm died down, that the pain was still there, just the same).

In January 2000 I started the fifth edition of this book to bring it alongside its new stable mate, *Sarah Key's Back Sufferers' Bible*. The new book charts the decline of spines in a linear progression through different stages of breakdown but, even so, the same old questions still get asked.

The science of treating backs is slowly evolving but, as always, there are questions common to every sufferer, all of whom have a hard job getting answers. As we breast the new millennium, back sufferers everywhere still get a rum deal.

Anyone with back pain talks about it all the time. A vast league of fellow sufferers share a grim sort of camaraderie about their problem. The grapevine is enormous with lots of information, and even more misinformation, swapped incessantly. Back specialists talk in elite medical language, and patients misquote the specialists. Back therapists are encouraged to speak in barely intelligible quasi-scientific jargon, and to speak to each other, never to the patients.

There is a veritable sea of inaccuracies out there about back pain – the worst is that it can't be cured. This book is based on the premise that more information helps the cure. Questions need to be answered because an illness diagnosed is half-cured.

My only misgivings are when anticipating the furore from rarefied, academic circles because a clinician (and a mere physio to boot) is having a go at unveiling the mystery. 'Evidence-based' treatment is the current vogue, which means that for fear of being wrong one tweaks the tail of the tiger when proposing anything 'new'. Little current research provides anything we therapists can use in practice, hence and all of us are saying and doing different things. The wheel of progress turns slowly.

You will find bits of the text are fairly technical. Unfortunately, you have no option but to plough through. It is simply not possible to discuss a structure as sophisticated as the spine in a series of monosyllables and pretty pictures.

Knowing all that, here I go, grasping the nettle and biting the bullet . . .

1 Why is Back Pain so Common?

Back pain certainly is common, but the fact is that backs are only painful if they aren't working properly. Pain exists for a reason. When all the joints in our spines work smoothly, there is no reason for pain.

If you wonder why it is so important for a back to let us know when things are wrong, the answer is simple: the longer that spinal function faults go unchecked, the more widespread the strain suffered by the skeleton as a whole. The role of pain is to bring faults to the forefront of our consciousness so they stand a better chance of being fixed.

An active, well-working spine provides effortless gross and fine adjustments in the stance of the frame to set the stage for all deliberate fruitful activity. If it isn't working properly, we are put at a physical disadvantage and *all* our skills become handicapped. Although we may not be conscious of the change, the most simple, automatic and effortless activities become laboured and require more energy. Subtle strains are stored up, and this means trouble. In its perfect working order, which is rare in reality, properly balanced muscle groups at the front, back and either side of the spine prevent it from deviating from good alignment; correct spinal alignment is essential for placing all the other joints on their best working pitch.

But sadly our sedentary way of life, with many long hours spent sitting, compresses the base of our spine and makes the lower discs lose their bounce. In addition, our activity mode is frequently flexed or bent over, so the muscle groups holding the skeleton upright become unevenly matched. Without us being aware of it, our spinal base becomes brittle; at the same time, some muscle groups get tighter and shorter while others get weak and elongated. As a result, the upright spine becomes inadequately supported. It tolerates shock badly and starts running out of kilter, with all its actions out of trim. Everywhere, joints afflicted by poor working conditions are jarred and forced to work at awkward angles. As the spine suffers impact, the segments grind and chafe as they begin their own journey of breakdown.

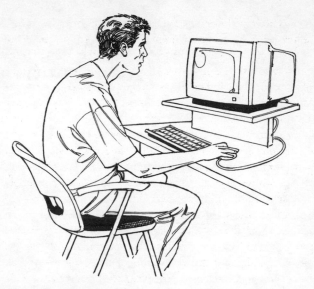

Figure 1.1 Much of our lives may be spent like this, crumpled over in concentration with all our joints bent.

Furthermore, because the skeleton becomes permanently kinked and constricted, we find we can perform fewer and fewer actions. All purposeful activity takes place within a limited variety of starting postures. We don't have the 'release' to do as we please with our bodies. We are trapped as if the wind has changed. Movements become stereotyped and repetitive, rarely allowing us the benefits from full, opening-out stretch. In fact, most of the time we are unaware of the delights of full, elastic freedom. Instead, we toil away within the same old patterns of movement. We put the toothbrush away, we open the car door; we might even go the whole day without doing one original movement. Day after day we grind the joints back and forth over the same old territory. Eventually, the joints lose their 'play' and become almost rigid except in its well-worn tracks. I don't have to tell you this is not good for them!

With this background of poor shock absorption and muscle imbalance, the working spine is debilitated in everything it does. The discs dry out and lose their romp, and the muscles and ligaments lose their stretch. The final straw is when we *do* decide to get out of that chair and do a bit of exercise; we do it with such ferocious gusto, we then introduce a whole lot of new and sudden strains on top of the older ones. The combination is lethal. No wonder such a high percentage of the population has or has had backache.

Mind you, there is a good reason why we are gripped by a sudden desire to leap out of that chair and fling ourselves into frenzied activity. It is a subconscious attempt to redress the balance. It is a desire to 'reflate' the spine, to puff up the lumbar discs and bump up their shock absorption; an intuitive yearning to experience the skeleton at full stretch. It makes us feel so good to S-T-R-E-T-C-H, to open out the frame widely and savour the delights of emancipated freedom rather than permanent, static flexion. This 'spurt' is our modern-day method of releasing energies once used in foraging for food and fighting off enemies.

However, unexpected physical activity can put a handicapped skeleton under duress. If you lead a sedentary life, sitting for hours behind a desk or hunched over a steering wheel, you can 'do something' to your back with unnerving ease. A history of poor posture and basal compression makes it all too easy to harm a spinal segment. You can then develop a simple linkage problem and so it all begins. Sooner or later, back pain will develop. Whether it becomes a nuisance or a nightmare, the fact is, if the function fault worsens, the pain will worsen.

If we are to rectify the problem and thus get rid of the pain, we cannot afford to ignore the fact that the spine is compressed and failing to work properly. It is useless to swallow pills or strap yourself into a corset. It is often equally inappropriate to operate on the link surgically and try fixing it that way; which is rather like taking a hammer and chisel to a rusty hinge in a door; when really all it needs is to make the discs puffy again. A scalpel cannot cut out stiffness, any more than a chisel can cut out rust. There is no object to be removed; *the problem is a function fault.*

The first steps in curing an aching back are persuading the low lumbar discs to reflate and making the stiff spinal segments work better. And here is the good news. The more the segments *are* moved, the more they *can* move and the more they *will want to* move. Working them back and forth gradually achieves a better fluid exchange, which keeps them more robust and able to rebuff shock. The link becomes more stretchable, pressure lifts off the walls, and pain starts to recede.

Different as our individual approaches are, we practitioners working in the field of manual medicine have thousands of patients who can testify to this. It works! This is what 'spinal mobilisation' and the rest of this book is all about.

2 Back to Basics

First, let's start with the basics, in our search for a cure for back pain.

WHAT IS A BACK?

The spine is a tall, graceful column which rises out of the pelvis and waves in the breeze. It is jointed throughout its length into twenty-four small segments called vertebrae.

Seven vertebrae make up the neck. Twelve make up the thorax, or chest part of the spine. Each of these thoracic (or dorsal) vertebrae has a rib coming off either side which encircles the chest wall and joins the sternum, or breastbone, at the front. The ribs move as we breathe in, like bucket handles, and with each in-breath, the ribs lift up and out as the lungs fill with fresh air. As we breathe out, expelling stale air, the bucket handles move down and in again, as if to rest on the rim of the bucket until the next inspiration.

By and large, the thoracic part of the spine moves less generously than any other part. This is hardly surprising when one considers the engineering feat in attaching a pair of ribs to either side of each thoracic vertebra. The ribs move incessantly every time we take a breath, and carry on doing so without faltering. At the same time, that part of the spine could be contorted into throwing a cricket ball, walking, talking to a colleague or simply turning over in bed.

Five vertebrae make up the low back part of the spine, sometimes called the lumbar spine. Although the lumbar vertebrae are very bulky and strong, and built to carry a lot of weight, they are also exceedingly light. This is because the bones themselves are not solid. If you were to cut one open, you would find it looks like a honeycomb inside. In reality, it is a three-dimensional grid of narrow, bony pillars: the vertical ones act like struts which resist the flattening pressure of weight from above and the horizontal ones act like cross-bars which prevent the vertical ones buckling. The lowest lumbar vertebra sits about five centimetres below waist level, higher than you might think.

4

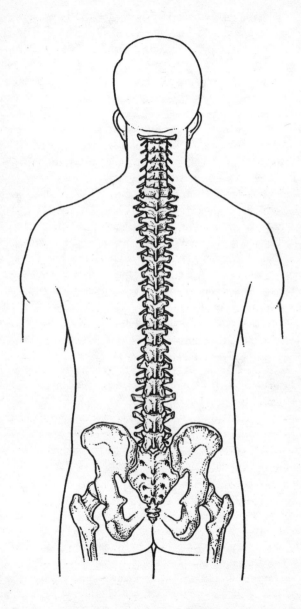

Figure 2.1 Posterior view of the human spine.

The base of the spine sits on the sacrum. This is a large, triangular wedge of bone which joins the two ear-shaped bones of the pelvis (the ilia) at the sacro-iliac joints on either side, where the two dimples are. The sacrum can be felt as a broad, flat bone above the buttocks and is made up of five fused sacral vertebrae. By 'fused' I mean permanently joined together so they do not move, except in a congenital condition known as lumbarisation where the first sacral vertebra is mobile (see 'Have I an Extra Vertebra?' Chapter 3).

The coccyx projects off the tip of the sacrum as a brittle extension. It is a vestigial remnant of a tail. If it protrudes down too far, it can be bent under with a hard fall on to the bottom or bent backwards during childbirth as the baby is pushed out of the pelvis.

In its upright state, a normal spine carries itself with all the vertebrae stacked vertically in three gracefully arching curves which are perfectly designed to disperse body weight in a balanced, effortless way. The lumbar spine hollows in slightly and the curve is called the lumbar lordosis; the thorax arches out slightly and its curve is called the thoracic kyphosis; and the neck arches in again in a cervical lordosis. As you will read, a properly functioning lumbar lordosis is vital to the health of a low back.

The vertebrae are separated by beautifully designed little cushions of fibro-elastic gristle called the intervertebral discs. They consist of a soft, squashy centre like a liquid pearl called the nucleus, contained by a tough rim of concentric rings of fibrous tissue called the annulus. The annulus holds the nucleus tightly corseted in the centre of the disc. Discs are perfectly engineered to bear weight by acting as 'hydraulic sacks' and dispersing pressure evenly in all directions.

It is worth dwelling upon this upright stacking arrangement of the human spine because there is an absurd belief that we are not designed to walk upright. Hearsay tells us it is a bad arrangement and we really should be crawling around on all four legs rather than striding about on two. This old wives' tale is one of many which clutter the understanding of human backs and shroud any cure with an air of defeat.

Even though standing and sitting cause squashing of the discs at the bottom of our spines, the alternative of slinging a spine horizontally between widely separated front and back legs brings on other problems, and four-legged creatures must accept marked limitation in functional performance because of this. Humans can get away with being relatively unfit and still maintain a more or less upright posture, but any four-legged creature must remain permanently fit, young and strong to prevent its spine sagging earthwards. For instance, overweight dachshunds with long-

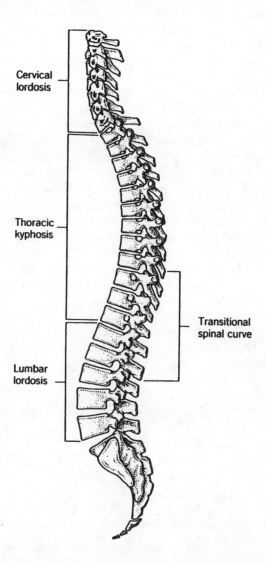

Cervical
lordosis

Thoracic
kyphosis

Transitional
spinal curve

Lumbar
lordosis

Figure 2.2 The human spine comprises seven cervical, twelve thoracic and five lumbar vertebrae.

drawn-out bodies commonly suffer backache.

Our superior co-ordination and balance mechanisms, combined with an upright spine, make it possible for us to perform many more sophisticated activities than other animals and the human spine has evolved in such a way that it can easily manage many different stresses. A horse can only go forwards quickly or slowly; it can never pole-vault or stand on one leg. And who said horses never get backache? There is a whole stable of equine osteopaths out there who spend their waking hours treating horses for ricked backs, especially the ones that jump fences or play polo. And those same horses might not yet be four years old!

By and large, a spine is far better off working vertically than horizontally. There may be hardening of a disc (which causes a stiff spinal segment), or even the occasional ballooning of one lower down if subjected to torsional strains (the 'slipped disc'), but these problems are eminently reversible, especially if caught early on.

The human spine performs three basic functions. It provides *support* to keep us upright. It has the *mobility* to bend and lift, and to put two long arms about; it adapts the torso to the walking process; and it carries an extremely heavy head which constantly nods and swivels during activity. The spine therefore provides dynamic mobility and support. It is also a

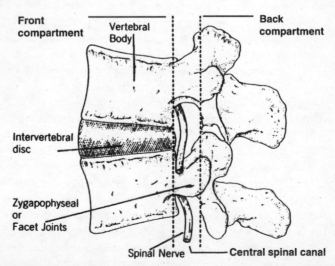

Figure 2.3 The front vertebra-disc-vertebra compartment bears most of the weight, while the interlocking facet joints of the back compartment bear little weight but 'guide' the movement. The spinal canal runs between the two.

casing to protect the fragile spinal cord, part of the central nervous system, which runs down the inside of the spinal column from the base of the brain.

Spinal nerves branch off from the cord and pass out of the spinal casing at each intervertebral level. They leave the spine through short, bony canals called intervertebral foraminae. These canals are created where the bony notches of two adjacent vertebrae come together and make a bony gutter.

So it is true that those small nerves, almost as soon as they have branched off the mother cord, go straight into the jaws of the hinge between one bone and the next, to leave the spine. Not a good arrangement. That hinge only needs to get jammed or 'rusty' and – watch out for that nerve!

This crucial combination, where a delicate and important network of nervous pathways is so intimately related to a generously mobile mechanical structure, can lead to trouble. It is a mechanical set-up which, of necessity, must be in perfect working order because nervous tissue is extremely sensitive and does not take kindly to being interfered with .

Imagine a healthy spine and its normal joints and you will see how easy it is for things to go wrong. If the mechanics of a spine go adrift then pain is never far behind. Each spinal segment consists of a front and back compartment, with the spinal canal containing the spinal cord between the two. The front compartment consists of the disc-vertebra complex where the disc is bonded strongly to the vertebral bodies above and below. So, as well as the vital role of bearing weight, this mechanism also allows the secure, strong movement of the vertebral stack careening about in all directions.

The disc-to-bone union is strengthened by the extremely strong anterior and posterior longitudinal ligaments. The anterior longitudinal ligament covers the front and sides of the round vertebral bodies; the posterior longitudinal ligament runs down the back of the vertebral bodies and, by covering the back walls of the discs, intercedes between them and the valuable nervous matter behind in the canal. Strong encircling ligament therefore runs down the entire length of the spine, encasing the round vertebral bodies in a strong, elastic strait-jacket which controls movement.

Behind the spinal canal is the back compartment which contains the apophyseal or facet joints. These are the bone-to-bone junctions of neighbouring vertebrae. Slippery, glistening cartilage covers the opposing bone surfaces and helps them slide more easily against each other. Further friction is prevented by the body's natural lubricating oil called synovial fluid. The two opposite bones making up the joint are held together by the very strong joint capsule, the inner lining of which manufactures the synovial fluid. The facet joint capsules are often referred to as the capsular ligaments.

The facet joints act as a bony 'catch' to prevent each vertebra slipping off the one below. Their role, therefore, is to guide or stabilise the generous movement of the vertebra-disc compartment so it doesn't go too far. The facet joints act rather like two small outrigger canoes stabilising the bigger canoe in the middle.

In a well-aligned lumbar spine, these joints hardly bear weight at all. However, when the back sits or stands with too deep a lumbar hollow – an increased lumbar lordosis – the facet joints are forced to take more weight. They are not designed for this and soon complain.

WHY SHOULD A BACK GO WRONG?

The root cause of most low back pain is basal compression from the spine being upright. The weight of the rest of the spine bearing down causes the lowermost segments to ride down, making the pillow-like discs lose water. To a degree, this happens in a cyclical way throughout every day; the spine dries out and shrinks, the longer we stay upright. It occurs through the entire length of the spine but is more marked at the base, particularly if we sit a lot.

Compression of the spinal base causes the discs to stiffen but it can lead to semi-permanent flattening, which is more difficult to reverse. If the process escalates, disc narrowing can be picked up on X-rays but, long before this, the vertebra on top becomes sluggish in movement. This can be the first sign of common, or garden-variety low backache.

As soon as there is any dysfunction of the lower back, the muscles controlling both spine and tummy also start working discordantly – and this is usually how a stiff spinal segment gets worse. Problems can go on occurring through either front or back compartments, or both. If the disc continues to break down, it might completely disintegrate, so that the top vertebra fuses with the one below. Alternatively, disc prolapse may occur, where one section of the wall weakens and the nucleus squirts off centre, making a focal bulge in the wall; or you may develop segmental instability, as the disc progressively loses pressure and the disc-vertebra union loses cohesion.

On the other hand, the segment may continue breaking down via the facet joints of the back compartment. They can become 'arthritic' from the wear and tear sustained by bearing too much weight, or by their protective role of limiting bending and twisting. Eventually, the facets can also become

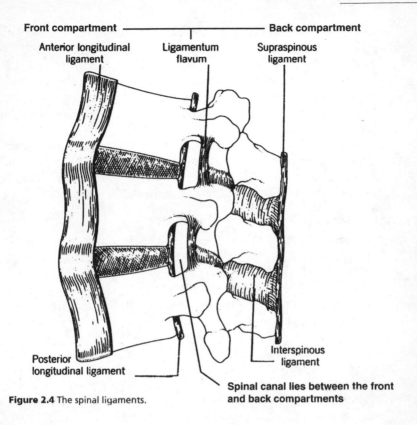

Front compartment ——————————————— Back compartment

Anterior longitudinal   Ligamentum   Supraspinous
ligament   flavum   ligament

Posterior   Interspinous
longitudinal ligament   ligament

Spinal canal lies between the front
Figure 2.4 The spinal ligaments.   and back compartments

unstable, either because their cartilage buffer has worn thin, or because
their facet capsules have become stretched and weak.

The human spine can be likened to a ship's mast. It has 'stays' at the
front, back and sides to help support and balance the spine. The tummy
muscles are the stays at the front and sides, and the back muscles are
behind. Laxity in any of the stays results in the mast either bowing
forwards, in the case of a slack front stay (weak tummy muscles) and an
over-tight back stay (back muscles), or the mast bowing backwards if the
front stay is too tight and the back stay is too long. The same happens if the
back (stay) muscles are too weak.

Balanced opposing muscle groups of equivalent length and strength
convert the torso into a mobile flexible cylinder, secure and confident in
everything it does and well able to uphold the integrity of the brittle column
inside. Unlike a ship's mast, however, the spine is jointed throughout its

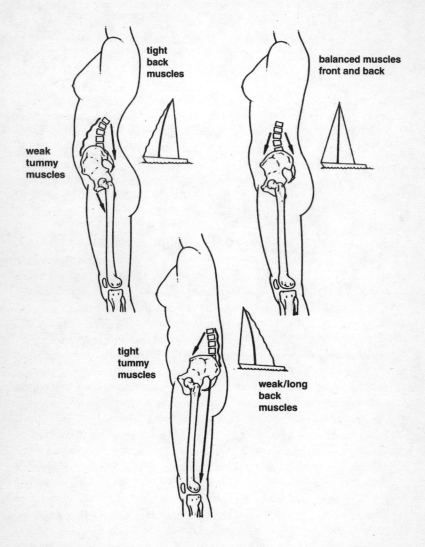

tight
back
muscles

balanced muscles
front and back

weak
tummy
muscles

tight
tummy
muscles

weak/long
back
muscles

Figure 2.5 The effect on the spine where there is a weakness of the stays which stabilise the column.

length into many smaller segments. A complex neuro-muscular mechanism controls the movement of these segments, all stacked on top of one another like a wobbling column of bricks.

The joints of the spine, like all other joints, have their movement controlled by muscles. Muscles work by contracting and shortening their length and thus exerting leverage on the bones across a joint. Each muscle group always has an opposing group to make sure that all joint movement is balanced. It should be just as easy to get out of a movement as it is to get into it in the first place. It would be very inconvenient, for example, if we could bend the elbow using the biceps but had no opposing group (triceps) to straighten it out when we had finished bending it.

A sophisticated machinery for co-ordinating muscle activity is working constantly as we move. So, as one muscle group contracts (say, the biceps), the opposite muscle group (triceps) pays out or lets go at a perfectly regulated rate, ensuring that the movement of the forearm is controlled and useful rather than jerky.

Usually, this co-ordination machinery works without a hitch and all joint action is smooth. However, every now and again we do something awkwardly or suddenly and jolt the spine, catching the co-ordination machinery unawares. The academics call this an 'interference of the co-relaxation phenomenon'. The vigilant, balanced interaction of the various muscle groups is caught off guard and we 'rick' the back. Usually the spinal joints, like any other joint, can cope with this kind of shock. The shock-wave passes through as a ripple or a wrench. Because the joint is healthy and elastic, the two opposing bones ride out the distortion force by shuffling about like boats riding at anchor. As the wave passes, they settle down again into their former, loosely-held harmony and there is minimal damage caused.

Sometimes, though, when this happens, one of the joints in this fluidly moving column gets strained. The reaction of living tissue to mechanical strain is always the same. If it is hurt, it weeps. A mixture of blood and clear tissue fluid called lymph oozes out into the general area and creates the familiar puffiness of recent injury.

Joint strain can be trivial. There is a quick tug and release of the soft tissues binding it together; the fibres are stretched but not broken and there is minimal swelling. At the other extreme, there may be a massive tearing apart of the joint when most of the soft tissues are ripped. Blood and other fluid pours into the surrounding tissues and there is a lot of obvious swelling.

Depending on how much fluid escapes from the injured tissues and on how much normal movement of the area is then possible (to encourage the swelling to be pumped away and reabsorbed by the bloodstream), a small residue of fluid will usually remain at the site of injury. Unfortunately, this creates problems. As the fluid lies there, stagnating in the tissues, it dries out and goes hard. It also tends to shrink with age, causing the joint to become confined by its own soft tissues. Mobility is lost.

The natural legacy of straining a joint is that it thereafter remains slightly stiff. In most cases you are never aware of this. After a period of normal activity, the movement works the joint free of most of its stiffness and you can carry on.

It is much easier to strain your back if you are unfit, because some muscles will be weak and others tight. Coordinated control therefore becomes slightly out of balance and less efficient in preventing strain. As I said, a joint mishap may not necessarily be major. It may be a fleeting twinge which quickly passes, or it may be a sickening, searing pain through your back. However, once the joint is strained, it remains strained. The spine stores the incident. The joint then goes through a normal process of reaction; it will be inflamed and sore for a while, then the soreness passes and the joint settles down again, becoming symptom-free. It will, however, remain slightly stiffer than it was previously and stiffer than its neighbours still are. This patch of stiffness is the core of the future back problem – especially if the injury caused ligamentous damage to the disc wall.

The stiff link remains. It need not be marked, just like a rusty link in a bicycle chain, or a sluggish key on a keyboard. For most of the time it happily participates with the rest of the spine in functional activity – perhaps a bit more slothfully than it should, but its neighbours compensate for its immobility by over-moving. Overall movement of the spine is not compromised.

All goes well until an awkward movement causes it to happen again. It is more likely to happen sooner if body movement generally has become distorted by pain. The new, awkward action unavoidably demands participation of the spine exactly at its immobile link. Because this segment is so stiff, it is particularly vulnerable to strain. And being brittle and inelastic, it cannot absorb the shock of the awkward movement as it happens. As a result, the already-damaged section suffers another strain *because* it is disabled.

The initial process of joint strain repeats itself, except that this time it is a little more dramatic and more inflammation ensues. A few fibres may be torn as the joint is wrenched, and there may be swelling in and around the different moving parts of the segment. If the spinal link is significantly irritated by the incident, the local spinal muscles may go into reflex spasm to protect the injured part, holding it rigid to prevent as much movement as possible taking place. The muscle spasm is painful in itself (as is any muscle in low-grade cramp) and it may be felt as hard and uncomfortable cords of muscle, like railway tracks either side of the spine. The spine becomes rigid and loses its gentle lumbar curve; doctors speak of loss of lumbar lordosis. When this happens, the pressure on the intervertebral disc is immense and the consequences can be dire.

Sometimes, if you have not heeded the signals of discomfort and have continued to do too much, the muscle spasm will go into overdrive in its effort to protect the underlying link. This effectively jams the hurt joint even more, preventing any movement at all – even though movement is exactly what it needs in order to start mending.

Conversely, the muscle spasm may become heightened if you are too inactive and remain rigid in bed, too frightened to do anything. The result will be the same, with the bones remaining jammed together and the joints (either disc, facets or both) getting increasingly bloated and stiff because

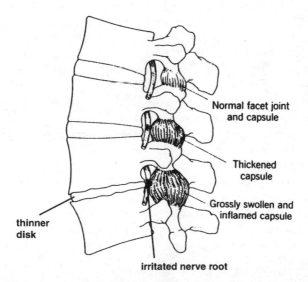

Normal facet joint and capsule

Thickened capsule

Grossly swollen and inflamed capsule

thinner disk

irritated nerve root

Figure 2.6 The progressive degeneration of a facet joint. As the disc shrinks there will be overriding of the two joint surfaces and puckering of the swollen capsule, which can oppress the nerve.

they are denied the benefit of rhythmic activity to get the blood through. Usually, guided by intuition and common sense, you get going again at just the right rate, after minimal time spent lying about. The joint soreness settles, the muscle spasm dies away and the incident passes.

If the muscle spasm stays severe and persistent, over a period of time – and I believe very much as a secondary development to the previously described process – the injured intervertebral disc, having been squashed by the vice-like pressure of the muscles in spasm, will be pinched out between the two adjacent vertebrae. The result is the so-called 'slipped' disc. Bear in mind, too, that the fibrous wall of this disc may have been traumatised over the years by the incessant torsional wear and tear. This will have weakened the strong, corset-like wall and rendered it more susceptible to bulging. But, when and if the muscle spasm relaxes, the joint surfaces will start to jostle and ease apart as the whole segment begins to disimpact. If the disc hasn't degenerated beyond repair, the bulge in the wall will disappear as the muscle spasm recedes and the pressure clamp comes off.

If the progressively troublesome link develops into a more serious complaint, the whole spine becomes progressively disabled. Eventually, you can do very little without stretching the sore link and provoking the muscles to clench harder. Both front and back compartments can then be continuously disturbed by routine activity, with permanent inflammation and pain as a result.

As a segment becomes less active, the disc separating the two vertebrae will start to shrivel; this is the collapsed disc or, even more emotional, the disintegrating disc. Discs stay healthy as long as we keep moving, but as soon as we start to lose spinal mobility, the process of disc degeneration speeds up. (You can see why we need to keep mobile.)

As a disc loses height, one vertebra sinks lower onto the vertebra below. The bony catches at the back of the segment override each other and the working hinges of the spine become even more jammed.

It is possible that a joint may become completely impacted, with one vertebra almost completely fused to its neighbour below, and very little disc between. This may mean that all movement is obliterated at that level and, since nothing can budge the joint, it is very hard to hurt it. This condition may even become entirely painless.

WHERE DOES THE PAIN COME FROM?

People specialising in the management of back pain have been slow to answer this question, perhaps because we, ourselves, have been confused.

However, we do know there is an enormous variation in the capacity of the different structures inside the back to register pain. Some cry pain at the slightest provocation while others are much more hardy.

Discs barely have a nerve supply. Remember that point! Only the outermost rim of the annulus of the disc has pain-sensing nerve fibres. A disc, therefore, can only be held responsible for causing pain if the fibrous wall of the disc is too inelastic to accept stretch or if it has lost its internal stuffing (water). Then, all weight through the segment is shouldered by the disc rim, just like flattening down the sides of a wicker basket.

Irrespective of whether a disc wall is emitting pain or not, disc walls often bulge. They are meant to bulge – they are shock absorbers. But more usually, it is the effects of this bulge rather than the bulge itself which causes pain. The bulge may press upon other soft-tissue structures nearby, which are positively electrified with a pain-sensitive nerve supply – wired for pain.

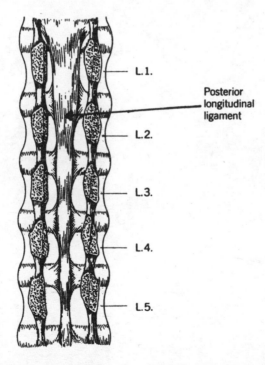

Figure 2.7 The pain-sensitive posterior longitudinal ligament is narrower over the L.4 and L.5 discs where bulges are more common.

Two structures most liable to be squashed by an unwanted disc bulge are the posterior longitudinal ligament and the spinal nerve root. Irritation of the spinal nerve will be discussed in greater detail later in this chapter; for the moment we will focus on irritating the posterior longitudinal ligament.

The posterior longitudinal ligament has an extremely rich nerve supply and it's very touchy whenever subjected to mechanical stresses or chemical irritation from nearby inflammation. It is easy for an unhealthy bulging intervertebral disc to painfully distort the posterior longitudinal ligament. Then you will feel back pain.

Interestingly enough, the posterior ligament begins to narrow in its width at the upper lumbar level, so that at L4 and L5 (the vertebral levels most commonly afflicted by disc bulges), it is only half as wide as it is higher up. It could almost be said that this is a careful design detail, since it tapers as it nears the site of most common disc-bulge activity, thereby reducing its

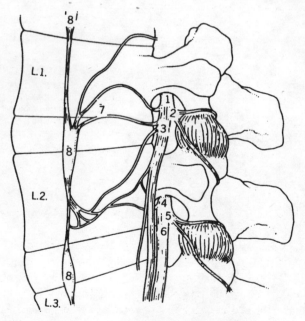

1 – 1st lumbar nerve	5 – Dorsal lumbar nerve
2 – Dorsal lumbar nerve	6 – Ventral lumbar nerve
3 – Ventral lumbar nerve	7 – Rami communicans
4 – 2nd lumbar nerve	8 – Sympathetic trunk ganglion

Figure 2.8 All facet joints are clothed in a complex interlinking lacework of nerves, 'wired' for pain.

exposed flank to potential injury. However, the posterior longitudinal ligament can also elicit pain when it develops adaptive shortening across a narrowed disc space. This narrow band of tightening can be painful when the spine bends and it cannot 'give' with the general stretch.

Other very sensitive structures inside a back which are commonly responsible for sending out pain messages are the facet joints. They are situated in the back compartment of each spinal segment as two sets, top and bottom (see Figure 2.8).

These little joints have a very rich nervous network which keeps the brain bombarded with information on how they are doing. If the facets are malfunctioning, their nerve supply reveals this in the form of pain.

I believe that trouble with the facet joints is the second most common cause of back pain. The facets are the easiest part of the spine to pull apart; their freedom is also their Achilles' heel. You only have to recall the astonishing versatility of this flexible column to realise that although its performance is generous, it is also vulnerable. Sudden or ill-considered moves can easily rick a facet joint. The joint then swells and goes stiff, becoming in itself an ample source of pain.

Think how distressingly painful a twisted ankle can be. The facet joints of the back are no different, except that they are much smaller and there are many more of them crowded into a small space, with a dense network of sensitive nerves threading throughout. When an ankle starts to swell and creak on movement, we really know about it. A sore joint in the back is just the same – except that the back is less precise in telling us exactly what is hurting.

To make matters worse, in addition to the facet joint being swollen and painful, its excessively engorged bulk may press on, and hurt, a nearby spinal nerve. This causes more pain, this time from both the joint and the nerve – a very common cause of sciatica (leg pain).

This brings me to the spinal nerves themselves, which are extremely pain-sensitive. They can be chemically irritated by noxious irritants resulting from inflammation nearby, or physically irritated by being squashed. It is not uncommon for a nearby disc or facet joint (or both) to malfunction, thus causing either to swell. Unfortunately, because the nerve lies so close to these trouble sites, it can be directly irritated, and raise the alarm of pain. And it is a pretty nasty type of pain, too. This is sciatica, or 'projected' nerve-root pain. Typically described as 'lancinating', it shoots down the leg in sharp, searing waves of agony. It is often associated with numbness, pins and needles and weakness of the leg muscles.

Another spinal component which is less commonly the source of back pain is the dura, that thin film of membranous wrapping which drapes around and protects the spinal cord as it hangs down inside the spinal canal (see 'Why is Sitting So Uncomfortable?' Chapter 9). Sometimes, with long-standing inflammation of a spinal segment, this membrane also becomes inflamed, simply because it is so close to the primary site of trouble. The legacy of inflammation is the same here as it is with all other soft-tissue structures: the dura shrinks and loses its ability to stretch. It takes little imagination to visualise the effects of a mobile spine being tethered from within like this. It is a problem. On manual examination of the segments, they often feel puckered in or bunched up, like beads of a necklace threaded too tightly on elastic. Any position, especially one putting the spine (and the dura) on sustained stretch, tugs at the dura and causes pain. Dural pain is very diffuse. You would have a hard job pin-pointing exactly where in the back you feel it. It might extend up as far as the shoulder blades and around to the front of the abdomen. This phenomenon also accounts for a patient's not uncommon testimony of headaches coming and

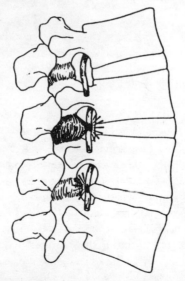

Figure 2.9 The delicate spinal nerve can be pinched either by a swollen disc or by a swollen facet joint capsule.

going with back pain.

Let us stop at this point to dwell on one very important fact: only a few structures in a back can be painful. Mysterious, even frightening, as back pain might be, its cause may be quite simple. More significantly, pain will always be associated with an abnormality of local spinal performance. In this way, it is possible for an 'outsider' like me to know where a back is painful. It always corresponds to the part of the spine which is not moving properly.

In fact, it is very easy for a therapist to manually feel whether an area of the spine is not functioning properly. It takes a bit more assessment and examination to deduce which structure in particular is causing the anomaly and therefore needs attention. It is also possible to tell if the problem is primarily a stiff disc or stiff and/or swollen facet joint. If the central core of the spine is stiff at a certain level, the vertebra sitting on top will be less mobile when pressured with the hands. The vertebra does not yield as readily as the others and feels like a plug of cement in a rubber hose.

Problem lumbar facet joints are just as palpable. We examine these by making a patient lie face-down, comfortable and relaxed on a couch with a pillow under the tummy to loosen the lumbar segments. You can feel them by probing deep into the back with the thumbs, about two centimetres either side of the spinal knobs – or should I say *can't* feel them. In their healthy state, facet joints slide away under the pressure of your approaching thumbs, and are conspicuous only by their inconspicuousness.

However, in their inflamed state, facet joints feel quite different in several ways. They are always enlarged or swollen. They may have a hard, brittle feel, exactly like a tough little ping-pong ball – indicating, incidentally, an older, 'drier' problem. Or there may be a softer, tense but squashy feel, rather like a half-deflated squash ball, which indicates more recent trouble.

If there has been a poorly functioning segment (front or back compartment) for some time, the tissues around it feel thickened and leathery. On initial examination of the back, the problem areas are immediately apparent simply by running one's fingers down the spine. There is always a slight 'drag' over the problem area.

A disc itself is impossible to feel because it is right around the front of the spine, beyond reach of the fingers. This means that the actual wall bulging of a problem disc cannot be directly treated by manually moving (mobilising) the vertebrae. When we do get results using mobilisation, we believe it is through loosening of the upper segment, as if shaking it free of the one below. Indeed, by introducing more mobility at the problem level, we help to 'lift' the stuck vertebra off the lower one, thus taking the pressure off the bulging disc wall.

'Slipped' discs, then, are only indirectly helped by manual intervention of the thumbs into the back, but swollen and painful facet joints are another story when it comes to the laying on of hands! The weary back sufferer, ensnared for years in a solitary struggle with pain, will experience a profound sense of relief when he feels, for the first time, the sure and knowing touch of experienced hands. From my point of view, it can be gratifying to observe. Not infrequently, I feel an outpouring of compassion for beleaguered patients, so beaten by pain. Meek and obedient, we are all children when locked in the jaws of pain. Time and time again, without demur, these desperate people unquestioningly offer up their wretched backs for us to have a go on. It is not difficult to see how shamefully easy it is for people like them to fall into the hands of unscrupulous practitioners who promise the world and abuse a sore spine sickeningly in the process.

Human touch is such a neglected balm. More is the pity, because it can be powerful medicine; so deft and sure it seems almost magical. Furthermore, thumbs are perfectly designed to delve around in human spines. Just the right size, just the right shape; if only sometimes lacking in force. For this reason, I sometimes, in some circumstances, use my feet.

Figure 2.10 It is easy to feel the facet joints.

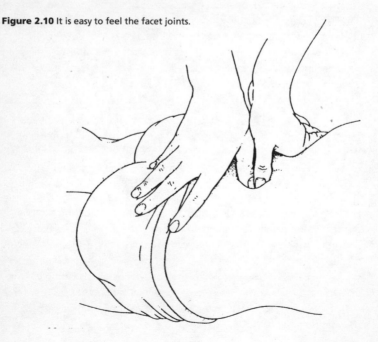

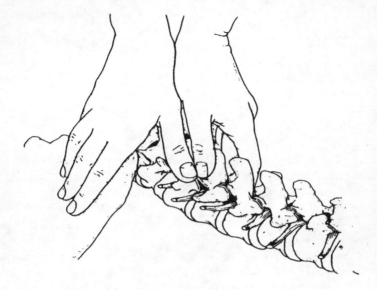

Figure 2.10 Feeling the facet joints – an internal view.

3 Diagnosing the Problem

Apart from their pain, back sufferers always have two complaints: one, that everyone is bored and possibly disbelieving of their problem and, two, they are never told exactly what is wrong.

The spine is an extremely sophisticated piece of machinery and in all probability, especially if you have been in trouble for some time, there will be more than one thing wrong at once. Every day I am asked the same questions. You patients are understandably very interested in what is wrong. And we therapists, who deal with bad backs in epidemic numbers, are in a position to make a thoughtful guess. But, bear in mind that our answers are only informed assumptions and one can never speak in absolute terms. Medicine is not an exact science. There are too many humans in it for that.

HAVE I SLIPPED A DISC?

A 'slipped' disc is not as common as everyone thinks, but when it does occur it is a most difficult problem to manage. A true 'slipped' disc often needs surgical paring before recovery can take place. But to describe how a disc goes wrong, I must first describe how it works normally.

Discs dampen the shock of spinal movement. They are resilient fibro-elastic cushions which sit between the vertebrae and act as buffers. Each disc is strongly bonded to the vertebrae above and below it. At the centre of each is a liquid ball-bearing, or spherical ball of fluid, called the nucleus. This acts like a hydraulic sack which disperses the effects of impact coming up from below and weight bearing down from above. The nuclear material is jelly-like and exhibits a unique ability to attract water to itself. This helps keep fluid in the centre of the disc when it is squashed, which in turn helps the nucleus transmit loads to its periphery. In the upward direction, the pressure of the nucleus counteracts superincumbent weight, and, thrusting radially, it stops the walls of the disc buckling under load.

The disc wall (the annulus) is unusually strong, but is also elastic. It consists of concentric rings of fibrous material, meshed together to make a tenacious circular corset. Each layer of the wall has fibrous strands aligned at 90 degrees to the previous layer, making a living lattice, just like the walls of a radial car-tyre. The incompressible duo of nucleus and lattice makes the disc unsquashable, like a high-tensile spring, thrusting the vertebrae apart.

The powerfully self-centred jelly sack makes for a rigorously stable arrangement. It means that the nucleus can never be forced, under pressure, out of the centre. If the disc is healthy (the big 'if'), even cutting healthy disc walls experimentally with a scalpel will not cause the nucleus to squeeze through. This fact alone disproves the popular notion of one ill-considered move 'putting a disc out'.

Nuclear material only squashes out when it has degraded. The fluid changes in colour and viscosity and loses internal cohesion. Under pressure, it spreads out inside the disc, thus placing extra load on the inside walls. This slowly pulverises the walls, making nicks and chinks in the inner layers through which nuclear material can burrow out. This whole process is greatly accelerated by repetitive bending, lifting and twisting habits.

The properties of ball-bearing centre and strong retaining wall make possible the spectacular mobility of our spines. They allow the vertebrae to sit on top of each other and roll around confidently in secure and grandiose spinal movement. It allows us to bend over double in order to do up our shoelaces and then flip up straight again, in one easy fluid action.

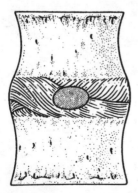

Figure 3.1.1 The wall of the disc is like a living lattice.

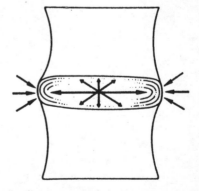

Figure 3.1.2 The disc as a hydraulic sack dispersing pressure outwards in all directions.

HAVE I A STIFF SPINAL SEGMENT?

Unfortunately discs are wont to degenerate, and the more prematurely aged they become, the more likely they are to cause trouble. As described earlier, as the aftermath of a previous jolt or wrench to the ligamentous wall of the disc, a spinal segment may tighten up and become less mobile. This is unfortunate, because a disc relies on full-scale segmental movement to help it suck in fluid and nutrients. With lack of movement it silently starves.

But even precluding injury, sustained compression of the base of the spine causes the discs to become flattened and brittle as we progressively squeeze water out. The predominant causes are excessive standing and sitting. In their compressed state, the discs at the bottom of the stack become poorer shock absorbers. They also start resisting separation whenever the spinal segments try to pull apart. This makes the vertebra sitting on top of the stiff disc sluggish – and this is what we manual therapists can feel from the outside with our hands.

One stiff link in the midst of a well-oiled chain becomes easier and easier to hurt, until it eventually squeaks and emits pain with every move the spine makes. The stiff segment can vary in irritability from faintly painful (when usually it simply feels stiff), to a low-grade permanent ache, to

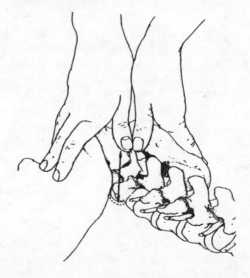

Figure 3.2 Pressure on the back of the spinous process will reveal a stiff spinal segment. It feels like piano keys which won't go down.

unbearably tender (when it is common to believe you have cancer). I believe stiff spinal segments account for an extraordinarily high incidence of simple back pain. A stiff vertebra may not show up on routine scanning (by x-rays, CT and MRI) but if you know what you are looking for, it is obvious to the touch. Most normal spines have a random scattering of stiff segments (most of which are not painful), but they set the stage for worse things to come.

Experienced hands can easily feel a stiff segment in the spine. From above (with the patient lying prone over a pillow) the vertebra is unwilling to glide forward under pressure and feels exactly like a piano key where the spring underneath is too stiff. As well as encountering postero-anterior stiffness (PA resistance), the vertebra may also be loath to swivel on its axis. Its backward-projecting tail may be free to swing from left to right, for example, but not the other way. We then say that the vertebra is blocked to 'transverse pressures' from the right. A previous twisting injury may have caused this; the vertebra twists on its axis and then becomes locked, just like the lid of a screw-top jar being screwed down. The art of manual treatment involves using the thumbs (and sometimes the elbow or the foot) to work a stiff vertebra free, at a rate which loosens it, without making it too sore.

DO I HAVE A SICK DISC?

A quicker mode of disc degeneration has been described by Twomey and Bogduk, leading researchers in the field of biodynamics of the lumbar spine. They postulate that the first stage of disc breakdown is a tiny fracture of the end-plate, the thin cartilaginous interface between disc and vertebra, the weakest point in the internal structure of the spine. Impact up through the spine (for example through aviators' ejection seats or hard falls on the bottom), can blow a small hole in one of these fragile plates. Although it may not be especially painful at the time, it has consequences later on. Part of the nucleus may be forced into the bone cavity, or blood may be forced into the aseptic heart of the disc. Whichever way, the trespass is seen as a foreign invasion and the auto-immune defences are rallied and the disc is destroyed.

As it deflates, the disc rim bears the brunt of the load. It may fast-track in no time from being a fairly normal, healthy disc to a stiff flattened one resembling a piece of compressed carpet. This soon causes a stiff spinal segment.

Sometimes the disc's breakdown is even swifter as it rapidly turns into a flaccid, gummy sack. It leapfrogs straight past the stiffness phase, making the disc resemble a rubbery spinal connector instead of a tense fibro-elastic sack. Clinically, this process is termed 'primary disc disease' although it is never an easy diagnosis to make. Apart from a deep central back pain, for diagnosis we have to rely heavily on MRI scanning (a black disc on MRI indicates a sick disc). The problem can go on to become a bulging or herniated disc, as cracks in the wall develop with further wear and tear. This can then cause leg pain as well as the original back pain. You *can*, however, pre-empt this stage with proper management.

Be warned that primary disc disease is not easy to treat further down the track. Sick disks are some of the hardest cases to deal with. Months might go by when progress seems assured, only to have a discouraging setback for what seems no reason at all. Sick discs flare up with amazing capriciousness, especially after sitting, when the back stiffens and assumes the characteristic 'S' bend when you stand.

In fact, sitting seems to be the greatest problem. The lack of internal pressure appears to make the disc rapidly deflate so that the spine slews around on it, like a car veering over on a flaccid, half-inflated rubber tyre. The disc walls then traumatise further and pain signals go out.

Mobilisation can help to some extent. Manual tinkering injects some looseness into the tightly held segment so that it can imbibe fluid and 'grow', thus relieving the pressure on the disc wall. But best results come with tummy exercises. They shore up the spine within the torso, thus reducing the burden on the sick disc. The increased intra-abdominal pressure from the sit-ups thrusts the spine skywards, lifting pressure off the disc wall. It's just like squeezing a toothpaste tube with the cap screwed on; as the grip tightens, the tube forces itself upright.

If this back seems like yours, then I suggest you read the section on exercises (see 'What Exercises Should I Do?', Chapter 6). A strong tummy is essential for the welfare of your back. In this section, I have deliberately emphasised the difference between good sit-ups and bad. You should aim to curl up, as you tuck your chin in and crease your abdomen across the middle. Try not to jerk up with a hollow in the low back. This uses the powerful hip muscles which inhibit effective pure abdominals work. It also compresses the low lumbar vertebrae and encourages shear.

As a degenerated nucleus loses its hold on water, it is rendered 'expressible' and can easily be pushed out of the centre of the disc. If, by chance, the wall has developed a radial split from trauma, it is easy to see how the unhealthy material can squirt through the crack and become a 'slipped disc'. Forward

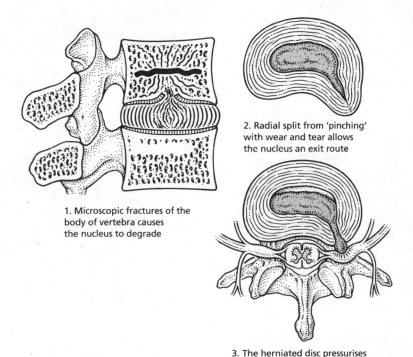

1. Microscopic fractures of the body of vertebra causes the nucleus to degrade

2. Radial split from 'pinching' with wear and tear allows the nucleus an exit route

3. The herniated disc pressurises and inflames the spinal nerve root

Figure 3.3 The story of disc degeneration.

bending and twisting movements of the body not only increase the pressure within the disc but can cause a crack to widen. This explains why it is often these very actions which ultimately cause a disc to burst – the last straw.

Whatever the reasons for gradual deterioration of the disc's health, the nuclear material does not usually burst right through the disc wall (the herniated disc). More commonly, it squeezes only part way through the multiple layers of wall. But the build-up of pressure in front of the straying nucleus greatly distends the remaining layers that are still intact. This is why you get your bulge (the protruding disc).

A bulge can squash other pain-sensitive structures close by, the most sensitive of which is the spinal nerve root. However, the notion of 'slipped' discs pinching nerves is undergoing scrutiny. It has long been acknowledged that pressure alone on nerves in other parts of the body does not cause pain. The funny-bone, for example, is where the ulnar nerve is vulnerable to pressure at the elbow. But, if you squash the funny-bone by lying on your arm, you will feel only numbness and pins and needles as it comes to life – admittedly an unpleasant sensation, but never pain.

It is now thought that disc bulges alone do not bother nearby structures unless that pressure creates inflammation – redness, soreness, oozing and swelling. And then you *will* have trouble. The nearby posterior longitudinal ligament inflames under pressure, and is thought to cause pain. And irritation of the spinal nerve can also cause either back or leg pain or both.

DO I HAVE A LOOSE (UNSTABLE) VERTEBRA?

Left unchecked, a flattened disc often generates wider spinal disharmony which can feed back into and worsen the original problem. Complications set in as the disc loses more and more height. The loss of stature leads to jamming of the facet joints at the back of the link, which creates more stiffness in the spinal segment and injects more trouble into the self-fuelling cycle. The muscles beside the spine go into a heightened state of con-traction, or *spasm*, thus increasing the pressure on the problem spinal level. Though the spasm is initially a protective mechanism to lock away the troubled link, it can turn a nuisance into a nightmare.

As the inflammation rises to a crescendo, the back grows tighter and tighter, thus exerting more pressure on the sick link. As the disc gets more squashed its wall bulges further, the local congestion intensifies and the inflammation escalates. A vicious cycle sets in. Eventually, you may be completely incapacitated by a crippling pain in the leg – sciatica. But even at this stage, if you lie low for a bit, and do some gentle exercises, the inflammation can die away.

However, when the fire goes out, the affected segment may take on a totally different character. Although not 'hot' any more, the segment may become unstable. This happens when the brittle impaction holding the segment together starts to disengage, exposing a potentially wobbly weak link. Because the disc has depressurised and flattened, the surrounding soft tissues have become slack, making it impossible to hold the vertebra in place. Deprived of a thick, juicy, normal disc to keep it tightly sprung apart, the segment can slip askew in the column.

As the crisis cools and the protective muscle spasm subsides, the tissues are decompressed, which eases the inflammation. But then the weak link is exposed and the back is vulnerable again for the cycle to repeat. It starts to slip around with normal movement which further stretches the binding ligaments; the tissues are irritated by the vertebra jiggling about and it starts

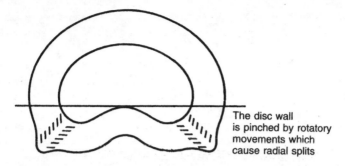

The disc wall
is pinched by rotatory
movements which
cause radial splits

Figure 3.4 The typical sites of greatest wear and tear are in the left- and right-hand back corners of the disc wall.

to hot up again. The back will go stiff again, often developing the characteristic 'S' bend (when viewed from behind) of sciatic scalasis, when one hip goes out to the side.

All in all, the back behaves in a very unstable manner and causes great anxiety, particularly if the possibility of surgery is looming. There will be increasingly frequent flare-ups, with pain down the leg and shorter respites in between; incidents which set it off will become increasingly trivial and attacks will last longer. The back will feel like a piece of board, stiff and sore for most of the time but interspersed with unnerving episodes where it 'gives way', folding up at the weak link. Even the simplest task becomes a chore; spontaneity of movement is lost. It is hard to say exactly how the disc behaves but I suspect it fluctuates between phases of flaccidity and angry distension; 'good days and bad', as the patients say.

You will find you can get by most of the time with a fairly rigid spine, as long as you don't sit for too long, but you will be exasperated by this rotten piece of machinery called your back. If it proves impossible to shore up the weak link by re-education of the small muscles holding the vertebrae together (your best bet) you may need a spinal fusion (see 'Do I Need an Operation?' Chapter 4).

As the disc deteriorates, the nuclear material sometimes bursts right through its retaining wall. When the pressure escapes, at the very least, the tension of the disc wall is released and squashed neighbouring soft tissues are decompressed; however, the nuclear material, by now toxic and a typical brownish colour, can inflame the tissues outside the disc wall, particularly the nerve root.

In either case the pain is considerable, either in the back, leg or both.

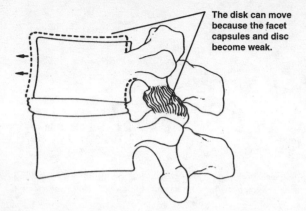

The disk can move
because the facet
capsules and disc
become weak.

Figure 3.5 Spinal instability is a common sequel to degeneration of both facet joint and intervertebral disc.

Being loath to stand on the bad leg, you stand with your knee bent, the low back pathetically rounded and bent sideways into an 'S', with one hip-bone protruding. (This is the result of the unequal contraction of the muscles either side of the spine.) It is extremely difficult to sit or to move about and if forced to make a journey – for example, to see the doctor or have an X-ray – you may be forced to lie down on the pavement, or the floor of the lift, to get some respite. You may have difficulty passing urine and you may also experience numbness and/or muscle weakness in the leg. The only solution is for a surgeon to decompress the area by removing some of the disc and then join the two vertebrae together by passing two large screws through the facet joints. Usually the results of surgery are spectacularly good and you will wake from the anaesthetic with none of that awful pain. A welcome relief.

HAVE I PUT MY BACK OUT?

As a practitioner dealing almost solely with problem backs, I couldn't count the number of patients over the years who have said to me: 'I think I've put my back out.'

The defence mechanisms which guard our spine are far too efficient to allow a segment to dislocate during simple everyday activity. Each disc is strongly attached to its two vertebrae above and below and cannot be dislodged with movement; the term 'slipped disc' is an absurdly inaccurate expression.

However, it is possible for one joint in the long chain of facets running up either side of the spine to slip slightly askew with a chance, awkward movement. A tiny slip of a millimetre or two (called a subluxation) can occur without the postural defences registering in time. Too late, the spinal muscles react to stop the slip and they clench with one massive spasm. This may jam the two congruent surfaces of the joint but will lock them slightly out of alignment. This is known as 'facet locking'.

The circumstance which leads to the facet joint slipping 'out of joint' in the first place is incipient degeneration of the interceding disc, as described above. This creates a depressurised link in the spinal chain, because as the disc degenerates, it loses water content. As its height goes down, like a hot-water bottle losing water, the disc goes flaccid and cannot spring-load its vertebra sitting on top of it as the spine tips. Thus the segment is more likely to shear. This type of problem is distinguishable from the one described previously ('Have I Slipped a Disc?') because the disc itself has no role to play. It has simply decompressed, leaving the facet joints to play out the scenario of dysfunction.

With repeated facet-locking episodes, the capsule surrounding the facet joint may become slack and unable to control fine vertebral movement. The facet is then solely dependent on vigilant muscle control to prevent untoward movement taking place. Alas! This is a tall order. Often they cannot prevent slippage with the most trivial, incidental movement. Avoiding someone approaching you on the footpath for example, or stepping off a kerb which was deeper than you thought, can cause havoc. There's an agonising jab of pain, right when you least expect it: the muscles were caught off guard and failed to brace you or, rather your weaker link, for the shock.

Sometimes the whole segment gets sloppier through incompetent ligamentous binding. It is said to be hyper-mobile and may become unstable. If this happens, you can put your back out with increasing frequency by increasingly trivial means; sneezing, turning over in bed, getting up out of a chair or car. The potential for mishap is endless.

However, you might present yourself for treatment saying your back feels disjointed, as if it needs to be 'put back in'. Almost invariably it hasn't been put out in the manner just described. Usually it is simply a stiff joint being stressed and then locked up by protective muscles.

The two different circumstances are easily distinguishable from each other. The acute subluxation takes place with a tweak or a cracking sound, followed instantaneously by a violent muscle spasm which takes your breath away and brings you to your knees. You become stuck in the movement, as if frozen in time.

On the other hand, joint strain of a 'weak' link can take place almost without you knowing. Characteristically, you will develop a stiff back the night after chopping wood or painting the ceiling. You have not put anything out – neither the joint nor the disc. You have simply strained the weak link in your spine.

The trouble with joint strain is that it suffers from the lack of a suitably colourful and descriptive catchphrase to describe it. It means nothing to tell your friends you have a poorly functioning joint in your spine and must hurry off to see your physio. But if you have put your back out, they will be likely to fall about with sympathy.

The best treatment for a weak/stiff spinal segment strain is to gently persuade it that movement is not such a bad thing after all. Movement is what it needs; gentle mobilisation with the thumbs, not another quick yank with a manipulation. Facet locking, however, is best dealt with by a quick manipulative thrust. This momentarily springs the joint apart and lets it 'clonk' back together again, properly aligned with its two congruent joint surfaces happily notched together.

A manipulative procedure with the characteristic 'cracking' sound has its single most satisfactory application here. Unfortunately, you can rarely get to the physio, chiropractor or osteopath soon enough, before severe protective muscle spasm sets in. This precludes the use of a quick thrust in the right direction because it will not allow any movement at all at the affected level. If this is the case, a good deal of time has to be spent relaxing the area and getting rid of muscle spasm so that it can eventually be manipulated. This may take days, but the problem will not be cleared until it has been manipulated. On the other hand, if you are lucky enough to get in quickly, though you may have arrived for the treatment bent over and locked, you can walk away on air.

As a routine practice, it is not a good idea to repeatedly manipulate a spinal link which has become sloppy through disc degeneration. Although one quick, delicate thrust may be necessary to unlock a localised jamming, any more than that will simply over-stretch the joint. It will become weak, with an increasing propensity to slip askew in the future. Although there may be immediate advantages in freeing the joint, the net long-term effect is a bad one: it further stretches the structures which are trying so hard to hold the segment stable.

With manipulation, patients often get hooked on a routine where they are permanently 'on treatment'. Their symptoms are real enough, but they are *being propagated by* treatment. It is not unusual to hear of people being manipulated once a week in perpetuity. Some blame (some only!) must rest with the patients themselves, because there are many who feel they have not been treated properly if they have not been manipulated. They are unwilling to submit to being mobilised instead because they feel it doesn't 'do enough'. Although the best approach may be to free the joint with the thumbs and then follow up with exercises designed to strengthen the segment, it may initially feel very passive and namby-pamby; just gentle pressure. I have frequently heard patients say: 'She didn't seem to be doing anything, just pressing with her hands!' Well, all I can say is: just give it a chance. The alternative may be permanent treatment, using techniques that keep you needy.

DO I HAVE ARTHRITIS?

Poor Western man, he gets arthritis just as he sits there. With his predilection for the sedentary life where so much functional activity is done hunched in stooped postures, performing a series of tasks notable only by their lack of variety, he stores up a heap of trouble for himself. No wonder. He develops a working skeleton regulated by muscle groups which are out of balance and of dissimilar ability.

It would be better if we ran around throwing spears all day and squatted in front of camp-fires instead of slumping in easy chairs watching telly. As it is, the unequal pull of muscles across the joints amounts to permanent wear and tear; arthritis hovering in the background. The joints fail to work at their best when guided by disproportionate control. Even in our most inactive moments it takes its toll.

Furthermore, joints that rarely enjoy the full excursion of their entire range of movement develop a reduced ability to carry out any movements they do have. The joints lose their freedom.

The great advantage of the living piece of machinery called the skeleton is that the more it moves, the better it moves; the joints respond and increase their self-lubrication. Movement keeps the joints young.

This fact alone makes it easy to see why therapy by movement is the only way! A stretchy, well-lubricated joint is healthy and will not give trouble (unless you injure it afresh with some other new incidental wrench or blow). The less you move, the less you *can* move; the more the joints dry out and the quicker they break down. 'Rest' is not the answer for arthritis.

Now, to explain this word 'arthritis' which worries everyone so! As I have

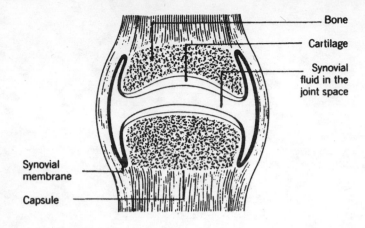

Bone

Cartilage

Synovial
fluid in the
joint space

Synovial
membrane

Capsule

Figure 3.6 A normal synovial joint.

said, all of us beyond teenage years experience degenerative changes in our
joints because of the limited ways we use our bodies. This speeds up the
ageing of joints. Then they are further aged by all the incidental jolts and
bangs they 'attract' during everyday life.

Prematurely old joints are too tight for their own good and extremely
intolerant to shock. This is arthritis as we commonly know it. It is simply
the normal ageing process of joints hurried along by the knocks of life. It is
not a 'disease'. It is simply wear and tear, and every joint will suffer it to a
degree. Only in its more advanced form will it be a source of pain.

Nearly all the important joints of the body are known as synovial joints.
These are just as you would imagine joints to be: two articulating bone-ends
covered with cartilage and held together in a bag called a capsule, the sides
of which are reinforced by ligaments. But synovial joints also provide their
own fluid so that they can self-lubricate. Looking at a synovial joint in its
healthy state makes it easier to understand the unhealthy state, when it
often gives pain.

The capsule is the sleeve of soft tissue which binds the two bones of a
joint together. The inner lining of the capsule is called the synovial
membrane. The role of this membrane is to ooze fluid, called synovial fluid,
which oils the bony machinery of the joint. Synovial fluid is magical stuff
which scientists have found impossible to duplicate synthetically. It's a pity
that some man-made oil cannot be squirted into all those painful, audibly
squeaking joints to ease their troubled toil!

Weight

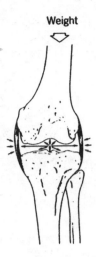

Figure 3.7 A normal joint acts like a hydraulic sack.

Synovial fluid exhibits the most astonishing qualities of lightness and slipperiness. When it is combined with shiny, smooth cartilage covering two opposing bone surfaces, it makes for the quiet, effortless 'slipping past' ease of the two bones working alongside one another.

The natural tension of the capsule and its synovial lining creates a hydraulic sack, by way of which a normal joint disperses the pressure of the weight evenly throughout, thus thrusting the two bones apart. This means, for example, in the case of the knee, that we are not actually walking on the bones and grinding them down. In fact, the bones barely touch; they just sort of slip and slide over one another, kept apart by the pressure of the fluid in the joint. The pressure is maintained by the natural tension of the ligaments and soft tissues holding everything together. That is why torn knee ligaments create such havoc.

Normal, efficient and effortless function of weight-bearing joints is further aided by the surprising plasticity of the bone underlying the cartilage. It can actually bend and absorb stresses much more than you would think. Bone is actually very bendable.

Things start to deteriorate and the joints become 'arthritic' when the flow of fluid into the joint slows to a trickle, the cartilage and the bone become brittle and the other soft tissues – ligaments, tendons and muscles – dry out and lose stretch. The bone loses its give and take and the cartilage becomes damaged by acting as a buffer in front of an unyielding mass. The cartilage becomes

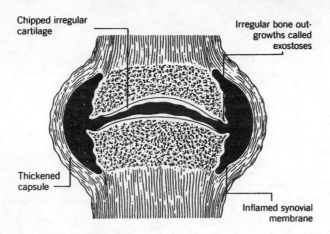

Figure 3.8 An arthritic synovial joint.

chipped and irregular, and weight-bearing through the joint becomes uneven.

As a result of uneven weight distribution, abnormal bony outgrowths form around the edges of the joint. These are called 'exostoses' and they never fail to alarm patients when they see them on their X-rays. Joints become swollen as synovial fluid pours into the joint space carrying large cartilage-eating cells. These are liberated to devour the debris of cartilage fragments which have been eroded off the main bed. Without this constant clean-up operation, the joint would soon clog up with grit.

However, there is a conundrum here because the very presence of the excess fluid engorges the joint and can be another source of pain. It creates a tricky balance in the management of any arthritic joint: in the process of making it run more freely (by mobilising the roughened cartilage surfaces against each other to smooth them and lessen their friction) we also have to empty it of the extra swelling this invokes.

When osteo-arthritis is painful in the acute phase, most of the pain comes from the fluid trapped in the joint. The joint (say a knee) often feels tense and hot, possibly from the overactivity of the synovial membrane in clean-up mode.

In the chronic phase of arthritis, it is harder to say exactly what causes most pain. It does not come necessarily from bony changes, even those unsightly knobbles you can see on x-ray. Having said that, it will come from the bone where the cartilage has worn away completely, revealing bloody, honeycomb-like bone underneath (a common condition of the head of the hip bone which you see in hip replacement operations). This gives a typical gnawing pain which is often worse at night and also with activity.

With most chronic arthritic conditions, the pain comes from two separate sources: mechanical irritation and chemical irritation of the tissues *surrounding* the joint.

Mechanical irritation arises when the soft tissues binding a joint together are stretched. This happens in an acute condition while the joint is swollen and the soft tissues of the joint are pulled tense by the fluid trapped inside. It also happens in older, chronic conditions when a joint cannot 'give' with movement. Everyday movement can provoke a stretch in a tight capsule and produce pain. It is different from the gnawing pain mentioned earlier; it is more of a 'stretch pain'. As range shrinks, so as not to provoke the stretch, all movement of the joint diminishes. You often see people with arthritic hips waddling along like penguins, with hardly enough range to put one foot past the other.

Chemical irritation is different. Pain in this case comes from the irritating effects of what we call 'inflammatory products'. Inflammation of living tissue happens routinely when tissue is subjected to trauma or disease. Wherever there is inflammation, substances are liberated which, by their presence alone, irritate nerve endings and register as pain. This is called chemical irritation and it explains how inflammation – without the mechanical component – creates pain.

The good news about arthritis is that it is much more rectifiable than you might think. It is not possible to do a great deal to reverse gross bony changes, but they were not causing much pain anyway. It is possible however, by simple movement, to smooth off chipped cartilage and pump unwanted fluid from a joint. This immediately renders it much less painful. Movement also rejuvenates tired, old soft tissues around a joint and makes them much more elastic.

Movement also speeds up the rather stately regeneration of joint cartilage. The marked pressure changes of full, end-of-range weight-bearing activities dints and releases the cartilage, thus creating a kind of circulation through its bloodless depths. Synovial fluid is pressed or squeezed through the cartilage, like water through a sponge, as the opposing bone rolls over it. It pushes synovial fluid into parts hitherto unreached, nourishing the cartilage and stimulating new growth from below.

At the same time, the gristly old tissues around a joint which have thickened and stiffened with lack of activity are stretched and released then stretched and released again, as the joint undergoes all this healthy new movement. They have no option but to allow the movement, especially when a physio like me is pushing and pulling them around, and their activity can quite quickly become more streamlined as the joint loses its 'woodyness'. Eventually it actually enjoys moving again and jarring pain becomes a thing of the past.

Most people think if it hurts, rest it. People are often unduly nervous of making things worse (even we physios are terrified of being labelled as dangerous). Patients carefully nurse their stiff and painful joints, slowly but surely making things worse. Incidentally, good treatment often makes things worse in the short term (see 'Can Treatment Make Me Worse?').

Of course, I don't recommend you fling yourself about with gusto as soon as you feel pain, but at least you should keep going and not grind to a halt. Often it was doctors who recommended rest; it was they who originally propagated the view of 'rest as the panacea' for all physical ailments. Too often, they would advise an arm should go into a sling, an ankle into plaster or a back into bed, when what it needed was gentle, progressive movement. You must remember that movement is therapeutic. The free, smooth, rhythmic action reduces swelling and thickening of the soft-tissue clothing a joint, and movement thus becomes progressively easier.

We manual therapists are in the business of making old joints younger. Our professional skills lie in 'bringing a joint on' at the right rate, but not in pushing a sick one too hard before it can take it.

It must be said, there are some cases of severe and recent joint injury (that is, trauma – the opposite end of the spectrum to the slow, insidious, degenerative changes of osteo-arthritis) where rest is needed; a brief, initial period of calm – between six and twelve hours – but only if it has been very badly wrenched and is still bleeding into the tissues. You can tell it is still bleeding if the joint becomes increasingly painful. It becomes tenser and tighter as more fluid collects, and often feels hot to the touch. Usually bleeding stops within twenty minutes, and thereafter movement should start. Then the sore joint must be coaxed through its first painful, tremulous movement. Nature only needs a nudge and it continues the process with increasing ease.

I HAVE RHEUMATOID ARTHRITIS BUT CAN YOU HELP ME?

Rheumatoid arthritis can be an appallingly relentless disease involving permanent pain and the disability of several joints. In this way, it is altogether different from osteo-arthritis, which is much more manageable, possibly affecting only one joint, and easily stopped in its early stages.

But there is some good news for the rheumatoid arthritic. It concerns the 'acquired' elements of the joints' affliction. As described previously, osteo-arthritis is caused by *damage* to the joints, whether by protracted postural strain or a one-off incident like breaking a leg. In either case, the joint is discommoded, and over time the strain tells, hastening ageing and ultimately the joint's demise.

However, with rheumatoid disease, inflammation itself may be the factor making the joint run badly in the first place. We do not really have the full picture on rheumatoid arthritis but evidence suggests it is caused by a disturbance of the body's immune system which creates widespread 'internal inflammation'. The result is the joints hurt. In severe cases, they are hot and even noisy when they move. Patients instinctively learn to adopt 'antalgic' (pain-relieving) postures, which bring some respite from the agony. For instance, they will know the best position in which to sleep: gently on the side and bolstered by pillows, with all the joints – knees, hips, shoulders, elbows and fingers – slightly bent in their mid-position.

Their restricted variety of actions, combined with a tendency to stay within the safety of these antalgic postures, means that rheumatoid skeletons barely move, and become increasingly crippled by their silent search for comfort. Unlike someone suffering from incipient osteo-arthritis, who is trapped by bad habits, the rheumatoid skeleton is first trapped by pain, and subsequently crippled by pain. Pain leads to bad postures, which lead to more pain.

The pattern of the illness is always one of acute phases fading into chronic or less angry bouts. Each successive 'bad phase' leaves the joints more and more bent, the recent acquisitions of deformity super-imposing themselves on previous ones. A lot of pain comes from these twisted joints. Admittedly, some of it comes from the pure inflammation of the disease itself, but some also comes from the acquired malfunctionings of the joints – an element which, with vigilant attention, can be controlled. As soon as the acute phase is over, the changes must be redressed.

Each wracking grimace of the joints must be tenderly released before the next real attack, or functional disorder will superimpose itself upon inflammatory disorder and deterioration will be swift. We must catch the contractures before they become fixed. This means stretching those joints; opening them out. Daily. It will be uncomfortable but well worth the price. Effective management of acute flare-ups always involves the administration of radical drugs including anti-inflammatories, gold injections or cortisone. You may also have physiotherapy to help straighten the limbs or, better still,

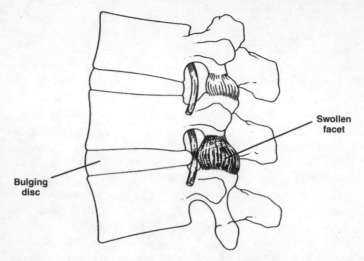

Swollen
facet

Bulging
disc

Figure 3.9 Sciatica is brought about by irritation of a spinal nerve either by the facet joint or the disc.

yoga, if you can cope with its zeal (see 'Sport And The Back', Chapter 7).

Rest has always played a prominent role in the short-term management of rheumatoids. But of rest and rest alone, I am sceptical. The best approach is joint mobilisation in combination with heavy drug dosages to control the resultant reaction. Rest, if you like, between stretching sessions. You'll need it.

DO I HAVE SCIATICA?

Sciatica is pain in the leg caused by a problem in the back.

At each intervertebral level, a pair of spinal nerves (which branch off the spinal cord higher up) leave the spine through a small hole between two adjacent vertebrae on either side of the column. The spinal nerves then pass to the legs to supply power to the muscles and sensation to the skin. Any structure that gets in the way and irritates the nerve root on its way out of the spinal column will cause 'sciatica'.

On their way through these exit canals, the spinal nerves pass close by the intervertebral disc on one side and the facet joint on the other. It is unfortunate, indeed, to have such a sensitive strand of nervous tissue running the gauntlet between two potential aggressors, either of which can become swollen and distorted by degenerative change.

The whole body is a map of different areas on the skin, the sensation (or feeling) of which is supplied by all the different nerve roots. The exact areas (dermatomes) vary slightly from one person to the next, but it is possible to deduce roughly which nerve root in the spine is being irritated by finding out exactly where there is pain in the leg, or where the sensation is disturbed. If the sciatica is very severe, numbness and muscle weakness may also develop in certain areas.

Discs have been blamed as the trouble-makers for years. If you had sciatica, it meant that a disc had popped out or 'slipped'. But how wide off the mark that glib diagnosis can be. This is just not the way discs behave. Discs never slip anywhere, in or out. They simply bulge and, even when they do, that bulge may be painless and harmless.

Thousands of clinical papers have been written on the subject of bulging (or herniated) discs – an average of two per week over the past forty years. I believe we in the medical profession have been brainwashed, and dared not stray from the given word. Remember that even medical people find it daunting to witness a fellow human gripped by terrible pain. And remember, too, that if one is placed in the position of taking charge, there is safety to be had in numbers; safety to be had in all espousing the same view. No wonder change has been slow in coming.

However, the general body of medical opinion is gradually changing. After enjoying an unchallenged reign for fifty-odd years, *the dynasty of the disc is dying*. Recently, one team of researchers formed the view that in approximately two-thirds of all operated cases of sciatica, the disc was *not* responsible for sciatica. These statistics are pretty astounding, especially since they refer only to backs which were serious enough to be actually opened up.

I believe most back pain is a simple linkage problem. There is too much talk of discs bulging and herniating. Discs rarely press on nerves to cause sciatica. It is far more likely a nerve is being subjected to pressure from an angry, swollen facet joint sitting right beside the spinal nerve.

I also believe that medicos have been slow to appreciate the true worth of manual treatment for backs. It seems something as 'low-tech' as stiff links, so easily located by experienced hands, and so readily loosened by them also, is just too uncomplicated for words! It has to be something more high-powered than that. We *are* in the space age, after all.

So often when you meet a patient, he holds his back, telling you exactly where the site of trouble is, and that it will be comforted by the 'laying on of hands'. He may be *using his hands* to rub his back in order to gain relief. When expert thumbs home in on that sore joint, he is surprised to have the problem so quickly pinpointed and giving that characteristic sweet pain. People exclaim, 'That's the spot!' Relief is, literally, at hand.

Another part of the disc myth ripe for junking is the belief that discs suddenly 'slip' out of the blue. The common claim is: 'I was bending over to pick something up and the disc moved out of the spine and pinched the nerve again.' Problem disc bulges never occur quickly. They take forever.

Healthy discs are extremely robust and inert. They only start bulging after they have been weakened by years of degeneration. Scientifically-controlled experiments where healthy spines of cadavers were progressively subjected to weight-loading eventually crushed the vertebrae to a bony rubble, while the good old discs remained sitting up as good as new, with no bulges.

Discs never sit there like a stack of upside-down saucers waiting for one to slip out with an ill-chosen move. Many people mislead themselves into believing their problem disc pops in and out at whim. Discs are extremely strongly attached; indeed, they are embedded into the bone of the vertbrae between which they sit, so one never slides out from between the bones like a dislodged washer.

Apart from sciatic pain, another type of pain can occur in the leg. It occurs in the same distribution as sciatica, but is 'referred' pain, not sciatica proper. The difference is academic. As a sufferer, you do not much care what is causing that pain in your leg. You just want to get rid of it.

One example of referred pain is a heart attack. The brain misinterprets where the messages of alarm are coming from. Pain in the heart may be felt in the left arm and up into the neck and jaw – whereas in fact the trouble is nowhere near.

Referred leg pain associated with back trouble is not brought about by direct irritating pressure on the sciatic nerve roots. The mechanism which brings about referred pain is probably as follows:

When a spinal facet joint is inflamed and painful (because it is in trouble), its own nerve supply picks up the messages of pain. This is felt as pain beside the spine and is a very common form of backache. However, it is possible that other structures, sharing the same nerve supply, will also feel pain. You may, for instance, have a vague, nagging pain in your leg that is quite far from the lower back. However, the problem in your back is the root cause and the pain in your leg is simply the real problem's effect.

You perceive the leg to be painful because the skin at that point shares its nerve supply with the area in the back where the real problem lies. However, the skin has a much 'richer' nerve supply than the back joint, so the brain, in error, assumes the leg to be the main source of concern. In the jargon of academics, referred pain is experienced in that part of the body 'with the greatest receptor density'.

It would be fair to say that all of us in the profession are pretty vague about pain, particularly referred pain. There is a lot we do not understand, especially phenomena such as referred tenderness.

The other problem which can complicate an already complex case is that, after a lengthy period of time spent suffering referred pain, the structures underlying the painful area, far removed from the source of the trouble, will eventually themselves start functioning badly and become a source of pain. This happens because we unwittingly attempt to spare that part of the body from too much activity. We reduce our demands on the underlying part, or use it awkwardly, which ultimately causes it to function poorly, and results in pain.

Not uncommonly, a patient will tell me he has a pain in the hip, and, although I will always check the hip – which may indeed show signs of minimal dysfunction, and may possibly be responsible for some of the pain – invariably the real problem is in the back.

Referred pain is a curious phenomenon, but it is distinguishable from sciatic pain – firstly, because it is more vague in nature, with less defined boundaries and, secondly, because the sciatic nerve will not be sensitive to stretch. Inflamed nervous tissue is very sensitive to being stretched. But if it is referred leg pain and not pure 'sciatica', the nerve itself will not be sensitive.

If it is pure sciatica, the nerve itself *will* be highly irritable and will be more than usually sensitive to stretching. To find out the state of play of the nerve, the leg must be raised off the bed straight, to as close to ninety degrees as possible. With severe irritability, the leg will barely get off the bed before there is an agonising jolt of pain. Stretching the nerve even to the slightest degree aggravates it.

With referred leg pain, this classical 'straight leg raise' is painless. The nerve itself is not directly involved in the inflammatory process and is therefore not in the least bit touchy.

IS IT MY SACRO-ILIAC JOINT?

Most probably not.

There was a time when the twisted sacro-iliac or the twisted pelvis was definitely in vogue. Everybody had one. Every vague pain from the small toe to the navel was attributed to bad goings-on in this joint. However, with

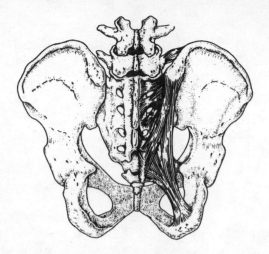

Figure 3.10 The sacro-iliac joints join the base of the spine to the pelvis. They are bound together by a tenacious criss-crossing lattice of ligament.

better diagnostic techniques developed in recent years, we now see things differently.

If anything is to go wrong with the low lumbar area, it is far more likely to be the spine than either sacro-iliac joint. Even with all that repetitive, poorly controlled bending we do each day – bad bending with shearing strains across the lower spinal segments – the sacro-iliac joints get by largely unstressed. And why should they complain? The back does all the work. The two sacro-iliac joints bind the pelvis to the sacrum at the base of the spine where the two dimples can be seen at the bottom of the back. They are fantastically strong, bound front and back with powerful inelastic ligaments which allow only the smallest degree of movement of the pelvis, rather like the unwilling 'give' of a plastic washing-up bowl. It is far more difficult to strain these two joints than it is the spine; that tall willowy column rising out of the pelvis, so vulnerable to misadventure.

In medicine there is a saying: 'common things are common'. In this instance, it is far more likely for a fragile little lumbar joint to be hurt by an accidental jolt than one of the large sacro-iliac unions, set so secure and bound-up, deep within the pelvis. However, there are times when a sacro-iliac joint can get strained. It is, as we have seen, hardly likely to happen incidentally. Rather, the accident must be fairly dramatic; a sitting-down fall on to the bottom, especially if one sitting bone (ischium) hits the

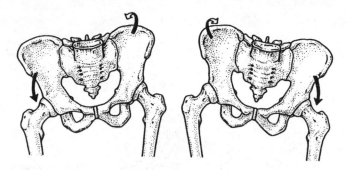

Figure 3.11 Twisting strains of either side of the pelvis around a central fixed sacrum.

ground sooner than the other, or perhaps a Rugby scrum collapsing on the man underneath (e.g., in a case where the player is already bent forward, so that his spine, being fully curled, is relatively stable, and therefore the sacro-iliac joint is the structure to go).

A sacro-iliac joint can also be strained when one leg is shorter than the other by at least one centimetre (see 'What is the Short Leg Syndrome?' later in this chapter). This is a more subtle type of strain which comes on slowly after many years. The joint complains when one hip is higher than the other because there is an unequal sharing of the body's load.

Strain is brought about by a twisting action of either side of the pelvis, either forwards-and-down, or upwards-and-back around the sacrum in the middle, which does not move.

The treatment of a strained sacro-iliac joint is just the same as any other joint. The legacy of strain is stiffness so the joint will be loath to move in one or more of its directions. To treat the joint and get rid of the pain, you need to find which direction it won't go – and then gently persuade it to go there. Find the stiffness and unstiffen it.

Osteopaths like to talk about displacement forwards or backwards, and how it is necessary to correct misalignment – usually with hefty manipulations to force it into a more pleasing anatomical position. I feel this is the 'ideal' rather than the 'real' approach. We manual therapists see the problem differently. We correct the 'movement blockage' and then let it find its right position in its own time – which it will do if it is not manhandled too much.

We generally loosen the half-pelvis so that it is freer to move any way it chooses. As a natural follow-on from this, any displacement will realign itself spontaneously if it can, with the negative and positive contours on the two opposing joint surfaces getting together and slotting into place as readily as they possibly can.

It is the gentle rejuvenation of the tissues binding the joint, changing them from dry and tight to supple and elastic, which transforms a joint from a painful to a painless one. I believe the position of the bones is irrelevant. It is the stiffness which causes the pain, and any misalignment persists simply because that stiffness is not allowing it to return to its natural 'untwisted' position.

The manual techniques we use must be fairly hefty because the joint is so tough and immobile, even in its healthy state. I position the patient face down and then get my knee on to the prominent ledge of bone beside the dimple of the painful side. I then kneel up on it and 'trample' the joint underfoot (or is it under knee). I can feel it giving under me as it starts to move more and more. It doesn't hurt at all except for that typical 'sweet' pain, which comes when the problem is put under pressure and which always feels such a relief.

There is another type of sacro-iliac trouble associated with pregnancy which is not purely the result of physical strains of the joint. It comes about because the sacro-iliacs are too loose.

During the latter stages of pregnancy, a hormone is liberated which acts on the ligaments of the pelvis to soften them. This allows the pelvis to separate slightly during labour so the baby can pass through more freely during delivery. This loose pelvis can be painful and, by being loose, it is vulnerable to mishap.

After my second baby, as a matter of fact, I had just this very problem. Every time I stood on one leg to put on my tights, there was a definite 'clonk' and shuffle as one side of my pelvis slid upwards in relation to the other – but then, I had been pushing and tugging a string of patients about until the evening of my labour! The good news is that loose sacro-iliac joints gradually tighten up again in time. Mine did.

Sometimes – and we don't know why – this loose pelvic state continues and becomes a real problem. The best thing to do is to bind the pelvis together with a sacro-iliac brace, a four-inch-wide belt worn tightly around the hips, below the stomach, to try to pull the pelvis together.

HAVE I AN EXTRA VERTEBRA?

The human spine sits atop the table-like surface of the sacrum, the solid mass of bone that makes up the back of the pelvis. The surface of this 'table' tilts downward quite dramatically at the front, which means that, having originated on the sacrum, the spine must arch backwards as it rises out of

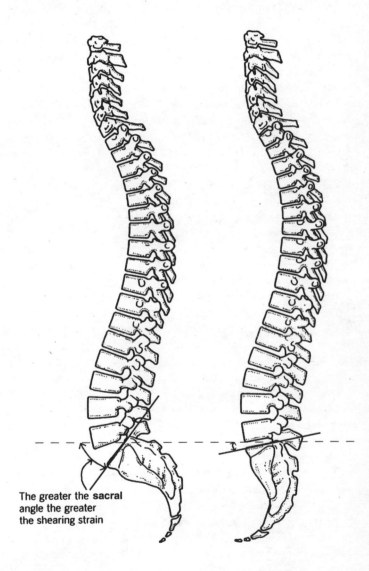

The greater the **sacral** angle the greater the shearing strain

Figure 3.12 The difference between a great sacral angle and almost no sacral angle.

the pelvis to bring itself back over the centre of gravity.

The greater the forward tip of the sacrum, the more the spine must double back, creating a greater lumber hollow (the lumbar lordosis). Some individuals have a sacral angle which is almost flat, which causes almost no lumbar lordosis, whereas others have a sacral angle approaching 90 degrees. In both cases, it can be seen how the sacral angle influences the workings of the spine. With too much sacral tip, there are shearing strains as the lower spinal segments slip forward off the sacral base. This particularly taxes the lumbo-sacral facets, whose role it is to hook the spinal base to the top of the sacrum.

Conversely, if there is no lordosis (or even a reversed lordosis, called a kyphosis), the central core, where the vertebral bodies stack up on one another like a column of cotton reels, cannot off-load weight to the facets. This will cause the lower discs to break down faster.

There are a couple of abnormalities of the sacrum which influence the activity of the spine.

In earlier evolutionary forms of the humanoid skeleton, the segments of the sacrum were not fused and, during activity, they moved along in concert with the rest of the spine. In modern man, however, the sacrum is solid. It is a rigid block of five fused vertebrae on which the upright spine sits.

The two congenital anomalies of the block-like sacrum are known as *lumbarisation* and *sacralisation*. Lumbarisation is where the uppermost segment of the sacrum, instead of being fused, is loose and participates, along with the neighbouring lumbar vertebrae, in spinal activity. The first sacral segment is said to be *lumbarised*.

Anatomists and clinicians have taken to referring to this additional mobile lumbar segment as an extra vertebra, which has led to confusion. There is no extra vertebra jammed into the length of the spine, but simply one extra mobile vertebra and one less fixed one.

The other congenital anomaly is where the bottom lumbar segment (L5) is fused to the sacrum, so there is one less mobile vertebra in the spine and one extra fused one. As such, it has more in common with its sacral neighbours than its lumbar brethren, so it is said to be *sacralised*.

It has always been assumed that such findings are clinically unimportant, but I cannot agree. Generally speaking, I believe both anomalies cause trouble, usually because of the incomplete nature of each one. With lumbarisation, it is rare for this additional joint to be completely free and, with sacralisation, it is rare for it to be absolutely fused. The pure extreme of both is not commonly found. Usually, the problem joint is neither completely loose nor completely

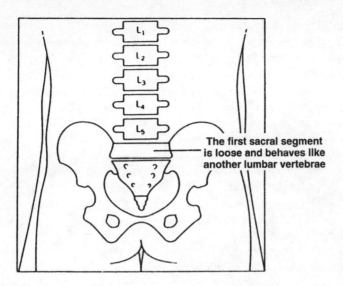

Figure 3.13.1 Lumbarisation.

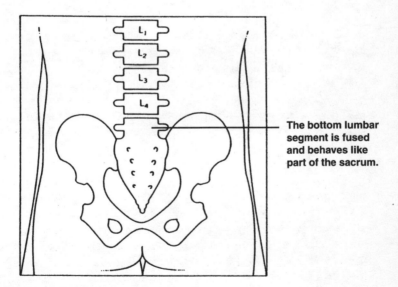

Figure 3.13.2 Sacralisation.

fixed but in a no man's land in the middle.

There is a certain safety to be had in a joint being completely fused, which helps explain the orthopaedic surgeon's penchant (though less common these days) for fusing problem joints. The rationale had always been – drastic as it was – that if a joint hurt to move then stop it moving. That this inevitably led to other problems in nearby healthy joints, which were sometimes as unwelcome as the original complaint, is another matter; the case for fusion can be clearly seen. However, if the fusion was not quite solid, everybody was left in a quandary. Indeed, surgical fusions which do not quite 'take' are the bane of the back surgeon's life. It's a good thing they are done so rarely these days.

Exactly the same is true of Nature's fusions. Those that are not quite solid are a problem. Using the analogy of an ankle joint: if you jump off a wall on to a slightly stiff ankle, you risk hurting it by landing heavily on it. The joint is simply not loose enough to roll with the punches and absorb the shock. It will be jarred and will swell and be painful. On the other hand, if the joint is in good shape, you will have no problem landing on it. It is flexible enough to absorb the shock and keep going. Conversely, if it were fused rock-solid, even though the landing might judder your frame, the joint would not suffer.

In short, it is better for a joint to be one way or the other, either freely mobile or rock solid, if it is to deflect trauma. Half-way between the two is highly vulnerable. Invariably with sacralised fifth lumbar segments, the fusion is not quite solid. In contributing to overall movement, like any other joint lacking mobility, the movement it does have is not good enough.

As described at length elsewhere in this book, the same scenario plays itself out where a poorly functioning joint sets itself up as an easy target for trauma. Strain heaps itself upon old damage, creating new damage and more strain. The joint's health, and consequently its function, deteriorates and results in pain.

I find exactly the converse is true of spines that demonstrate lumbarisation of the first sacral segment. Admittedly, that extra joint between the first and second sacral segment is said to be free but, in truth, it is usually not free enough. Again the spine is caught in no man's land, attempting to effortlessly incorporate this additional joint in its everyday function. Invariably, though, the ring-in joint is not up to the task. While essentially mobile, it is not quite mobile enough and is, therefore, vulnerable. Normal movement tweaks it, because the effort is too much for it to cope with. And, like the joint that is meant to be fused, it also gets hurt.

My solution is to get both types of joints moving – the semi-fused and

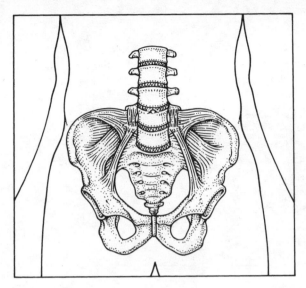

Figure 3.14 The ilio-lumbar ligament.

the semi-free. Attempting to get movement into a radiologically fixed joint always strikes my fellow medical practitioners as bizarre (if not mad), but treatment is usually short-term and highly rewarding for the patient. All the usual self-mobilisation exercises described later on can be put into action here.

Sacralisation also has another far-reaching effect, one not associated with joint mobility. This relates to the altered centre of gravity of the spine. It comes about because the lowest mobile segment is much higher, making the base of the spine less secure. Normally the spine originates deep within the pelvis. It is safe down there, anchored by a three-dimensional spread of ligamentous stays which fan out in a dense, semi-circle from the fifth lumbar vertebra to the pelvis, and lash the spine onto the sacral table. It is a masterpiece of design.

The most mobile joint in the spine, in terms of bending and straightening is between L4 and L5. However, L4 derives security for its flamboyant activity because L5 proffers itself as a sturdy mobile base. This partly explains why the lowest lumbar vertebra, L5, displays such relative paucity of freedom. It also explains why, when L5 has no movement because it is fused, the next level up, L4, is vulnerable when taking over the role. Though L4 readily compensates for inaction at L5, it does so deprived of

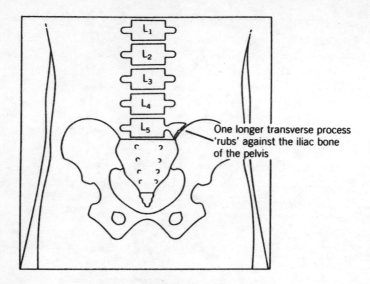

Figure 3.15.1 Unilateral transverse sacralisation.

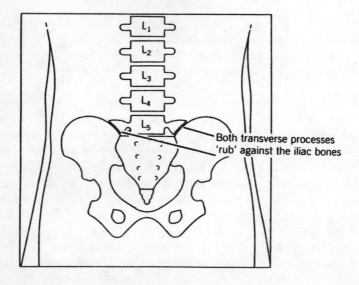

Figure 3.15.2 Bilateral transverse sacralisation.

the substantial ligamentous shoring afforded L5. In taking on the brunt of the movement, L4 is ill-equipped to cope. The flimsy L4-5 joint is then exposed to excessive strain and becomes over-used and eventually painful – a problem endemic to a sacralised L5.

Treatment of these disorders entails not only mobilisation of the fused fifth lumbar segment, but muscle strengthening of the union between the fourth and fifth lumbar vertebrae, not unlike the techniques used to shore up an unstable vertebra and developmental instability as a result of surgical fusion (see 'Do I Need an Operation?', Chapter 4).

In each case, overuse creates an incipient sloppiness of the vertebral link. This cannot be allowed to continue or the whole segment will become inflamed. Intrinsic spinal strengthening exercises must be brought in. Straightening the spine by unfurling it from the fully curled forward position will bind together the overused link above the fusion (see Figures 6.24.1 to 6.24.3, Chapter 6). As an exercise, it must be done at least three or four times a week, ideally after the rolling exercises on the floor, as described in Chapter 6, to limber up the spine beforehand.

Before moving on from this subject of sacralisation, there is yet another version of the condition which brings with it other problems. Every vertebra has several projections or struts of bone extending out from the central body. There are the two transverse processes out either side, and a single spinous process out the back (you can see these as the knobs protruding through the skin all the way down the back). Sometimes the transverse processes of the fifth lumbar vertebra are so long that they impinge on the two iliac bones (and sometimes the sacrum as well), either side of the spine. In this way too, the fifth lumbar vertebra is said to be sacralised. In this case however, the central junction between the body of L5 and the sacrum is fully, or at least partly, operative. The main obstruction to free mobility of the bottom segment is created by the transverse process grinding against the ilia with every move the spine makes. Nature copes with the bone-to-bone rub with its usual ingenuity; a false joint comes into being to lubricate the junction. Even so, streamlined movement is seriously hampered.

An even greater impediment to graceful movement occurs when only one transverse process is longer and impinges on the ilium, while the other swings free. Here again, the abnormal union is either semi-fused or, if there is more movement, a false joint comes into being. Either way, lumbar mobility is severely disturbed by this unilateral tethering. Every action is accompanied by a slewing-around effect as it tries to move away from the pelvis but cannot because it is unilaterally hitched. Again, the method of treatment is to release the binding nature of the abnormal joint by manually mobilising it to get more movement. This type of sacralisation is surprisingly easy to feel. As I probe around the side of the flat sacral mass, the presence of the false junction is obvious by its bony quality, almost as if it is just under the skin. With no sacralisation there is nothing to feel.

Investigating thumbs have no difficulty at all in sensing the degree of movement there. But, when it comes to getting it un-jammed, the thumbs alone are usually not strong enough. This is where the elbows come in! I use the point of my elbow with the arm fully bent, exerting pressure down the shaft of my upper arm. I direct the push laterally, against the ledge of the ilium, so as to prise the pelvis off the spine. It hurts but it feels delicious and it works.

WHAT IS THE SHORT LEG SYNDROME?

In a preceding section, 'Is it my Sacro-iliac Joint?', the shortness of one leg was nominated as a cause of chronic, though mild, sacro-iliac disorders. However, a discrepancy in leg length can lead to other manifestations of pain in the low back. This collection of findings may be called 'The Short Leg Syndrome'.

When the legs are of slightly differing lengths, the body automatically evens up the tilt of the pelvis by standing with the longer leg slightly bent at the hip and the knee, often placing that foot slightly ahead of the other on the floor. This gradually causes changes in the mobility of the hip of the longer leg, and eventually affects the function of the spine, too. Signs of adaptive shortening of the joint capsule and the muscles across the front of that hip become apparent as it loses the freedom to straighten. This process of 'flexion contracture', as it is called, takes place so insidiously, it can only be detected by clinical assessment; the sufferer is never aware of it happening.

However, inequality of hip freedom, especially in a backward direction, can have serious consequences for a spine, most markedly during walking. When you go to take a step forward on the short leg of necessity it must be of reduced length, as the hip of the longer leg hasn't sufficient 'give' to angle back sufficiently to let the good leg go forward.

The pelvis must twist towards the longer leg to compensate for the lack of freedom of the hip. This pelvic rotation creates a relative internal rotation of the hip of the longer leg, together with a 'pronation', or forcing inwards and downwards of the inner arch of that foot.

With a shorter leg, the low back must constantly adapt to the downward

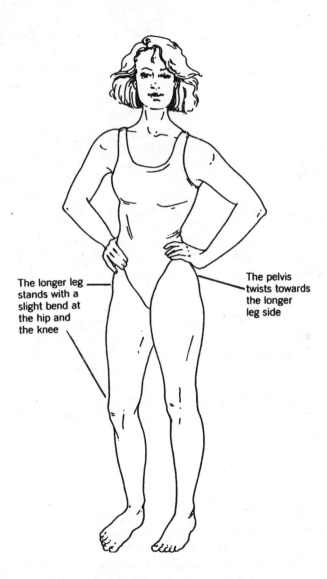

The longer leg
stands with a
slight bend at
the hip and
the knee

The pelvis
twists towards
the longer
leg side

Figure 3.16 The short leg syndrome.

slope of the pelvis towards that side. When the lower lumbo-sacral facet engages, it then becomes a pivot around which the rest of the spine swings. However, the anatomical alignment of the facets of the lumbar spine allow very little twist. Conversely, facet alignment in the thoracic region encourages completely free swivel (twist) of the vertebrae on their axes. Furthermore, the change from one to the other is abrupt. As the demand for twist comes up from the hips, the no-twist of the lumbar spine means these vertebrae move as a rigid block, until the movement reaches the thoracic spine with its different facet alignment. At this point (at high waist level), a massive de-rotation occurs. With every step on the shorter leg the thoraco-lumbar junction collects excessive twist, with the result that 'over-use' strain develops at high waist level.

The first step in dealing with this syndrome is to correct the leg length discrepancy. A cork or rubber insole is best, though only suitable for flatter shoes. This obviates the need for building up the heel of the shoe by the bootmaker. Women's shoes usually do need to be built up (because their fineness precludes an insole) but only the heel, unless the discrepancy is great. Under-correction is usually desirable. Scrupulously accurate measurement to the nearest millimetre is not necessary. The skeleton has learnt to adapt over the years and over-zealous correction may be too great a shock to bear. One simply attempts to minimise the difference.

The next step is to assess the relative freedom of both the hips, particularly in the direction of extension (the backward movement). This is best done by lying flat on your back on a bed, firstly close to the right-hand edge so that the right leg is unsupported and hangs down over the side (see Figure 6.16, Chapter 6). Hold the left leg around the knee and pull it as high up to the chest as possible. This will cause the right leg to move upwards correspondingly.

The tighter the hip, the higher this leg will lift off the floor, with a greater sensation of 'pulling' across the front of the hip and upper thigh. If there is no tightness present, the leg will not lift off the floor. Some hips are so tight they passively levitate to well above the horizontal. To compare this with the left leg, move across to the other side of the bed and repeat the action by hugging the right leg to the chest. Differences of freedom are immediately apparent, the shorter leg usually being much looser at the hip than the long.

This difference in hip freedom has to be redressed before the back problem will resolve itself. The best way to do this is to practise a stretch called the modified yoga lunge. If the right leg is longer, the corresponding hip will be tighter.

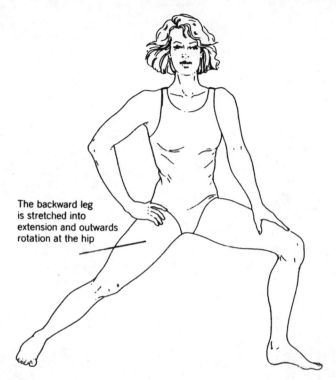

The backward leg is stretched into extension and outwards rotation at the hip

Figure 3.17 The yoga lunge.

So, take up a stride position with the right foot across at right angles and the left foot, about a metre directly in front of it, facing straight ahead. Lunge down on the left knee, making it bend to an angle of 90 degrees. With the right hip thus opened, you will feel a good stretch, which encourages extension and external rotation of the longer leg. Repeat three or four times daily. Take great care not to allow your back to form a deep hollow, because this stops your hip stretching fully. Keep your pelvis rotated well back with your bottom tucked under. Check the comparative freedom of movement by applying the same stretch to the other hip at least once each session.

Lastly, the spine needs to be assessed for mobility. It usually twists one way better than the other, the result of a twisted walking pattern over a long period. A therapist's thumbs can easily detect resistance to the swing in the vertebrae. There will be a corresponding lack of resistance when pushing from the opposite direction, as if the vertebra's movement is 'empty' or unobstructed. Full bilateral rotation must be restored.

To a certain extent, you can do this yourself. The best rotation exercise is done lying on your back on the floor, knees bent and arms spread out either side. When twisting the knees to the right, cross your right knee over the left at the knee and let both roll towards the floor. This will open out the left-hand side of the spine and also exert traction on the spine. Repeat the action to the left with the left knee cocked over. Roll several times in the 'tight' direction for every one in the looser direction in a ratio of 4:1.

The tightness of the hip of the longer leg also needs correction. Tightness here nods the pelvis down at the front so that the lower back forms a deeper hollow (see Figure 6.2.1, Chapter 6). This greatly hampers the self-stacking arrangement of the spine and creates shear of the low spinal segments.

There is another important reason why hip flexor tightness should be checked. Over-activity of the powerful hip flexor group causes reciprocal 'inhibition' or weakness of the tummy muscles, which are so vital to the support of the spine. This alone should be a powerful incentive to see that the hips get fixed. It is even more important, therefore, to read the section on sit-ups (see 'What Exercises Should I Do?' Chapter 6) since doing them badly will only create additional problems. Incidentally, no other exercise has the capacity to help or hinder you, depending on whether or not you do it well. Done well, sit-ups can cure a back problem. Done badly, they can cause one. So, in order to keep our backs in shape, we have to keep our tummies in shape, and in order to keep our tummies in shape, we have to keep our hips in shape. As simple as that!

WHAT IS SPINAL SCOLIOSIS?

The longer I spend treating problem backs, the more I find myself interested in the condition called scoliosis, mainly because it is so overlooked. Milder cases are often dismissed as malingering, whereas advanced cases have very little done except surgical correction. Quasimodo, the Hunchback of Notre Dame, had scoliosis, though to a grotesque degree rarely seen today. Scoliosis is curvature of the spine. From behind, instead of being straight, it displays an 'S'-shaped curve which may be shockingly marked or barely noticeable. In Quasimodo's case, his hideous hump, so cunningly re-created by the movie make-up artists, was his rib cage, twisted around and thrust up like a fin.

Today, with the screening of school children, together with better diet and heightened medical awareness, the disorder rarely deteriorates to the

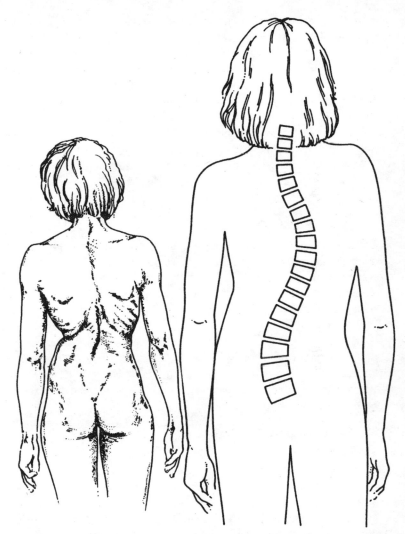

Figure 3.18 Spinal scoliosis.

same degree. However, mild to moderate cases of scoliosis are extremely common. Studies have shown that many people have a slight concave curve to the right in the mid-thoracic area, probably because of the predominance of right-handedness and also because of the presence of the aorta in the chest cavity. Moderate cases can be daunting, especially in adolescence, because they cause pain everywhere: headaches, pain in the neck, under the shoulder blades, in the lower back and sometimes down both legs. Families are often at their wits' end as no solution seems at hand.

Scoliosis usually manifests itself during sudden growth spurts. The rapid bone growth compared with slower soft tissue growth means the spine becomes caught in a web of its own soft tissues, as it shoots skyward. What starts as a transient, correctable hint of a bend quickly becomes fixed. Month by month, the deformity becomes more pronounced, as the child and family watch helpless on the sidelines.

With mild cases, the most effective remedy is vigorous sporting activity. Some formal side-bending also helps to 'undo' the bend. Yoga is excellent.

Countless theories have been put forward to explain scoliosis, although attention has always focused on severe cases. One school of thought proposes that cases of sub-clinical cerebral palsy can cause scoliosis, with its inequality of muscle tone on either side of the body. Such cases of mild spasticity are often hard to detect in children. They might be slightly clumsier than their peers, lagging behind them in 'motor milestones' – the appropriate level of physical ability for age – and this often worries parents more than any spinal anomalies.

Whatever the cause, scoliosis is often debilitating. Adolescence brings on symptoms with its inevitable growth spurts, the carrying of heavy school bags and long periods of study, hunched over books. But, depending on the severity of the curve and the amount of physical activity in one's youth, the strain of the curve may not make itself felt until later life when the elasticity of our tissues naturally starts to wane.

Normal vertebrae resemble house bricks. They have flat top and bottom surfaces with hard edges to maintain dynamic stability as the column sits upon itself and moves. The spine achieves equilibrium by self-stacking, with each vertebra exactly centred over the one below. Admittedly, muscle power is required once it shifts from the vertical but even so, the mechanics of the spine are a remarkably efficient, stable arrangement.

If the stacking of the spine is off-centre, though, it never achieves dynamic equilibrium. As it falls out of alignment, it slews around upon itself and bends.

In scoliosis, a distinction is made between primary and secondary curves of the spine, with the secondary curve (usually above) developing to offset the primary one below. This is a compensatory mechanism to keep the centre of gravity over the pelvis and, at the top of the column, to keep the eyes level.

Over time, this disturbed balance of the spine, first one way, then the other, leads to a plethora of subtle strains. As the spine tries to resist the bending forces, pain is generated by several factors simultaneously – the disequilibrium of muscle power on both sides of the column; the wedge-shaped vertebrae tending to slide sideways off one another; the strain of the restraining ligaments; the jamming of the vertebral hinges on the inner side of the curve and, in the thoracic area, the skew-whiff bucket handle arrangement of the ribs keying into the bucking and rolling sides of the thoracic spine. This may explain why patients with moderate to severe scoliosis have pain everywhere and why they worsen so quickly. Hardly surprising.

The surgical correction of worsening curves usually involves the distraction of the spine, as well as shifting the convex hump sideways or inwards. In my opinion, too little use is made of pre-operative mobilisation of scoliotic spines to optimise the post-operative result. However, with mild scoliotics, the combination of manual mobilisation and general stretching exercises to prise open and straighten the spinal hoops brings terrific results, both in pain reduction and retarding further angulation.

In cases of mild scoliosis, there is a lot to be said for unilateral muscle strengthening on the weakened side of the spine. Any all-round activity such as cycling or swimming which makes allowance for a weaker arm or leg (or one side of the trunk) will also be useful.

Gravity causes the half-hoops to bend or squash further so the segments at the apices of each curve are pinched in the bend of the hoop. On manual examination, it is easy to feel these jammed links. Due to the twist in a scoliotic spine, the individual vertebrae will always be semi-locked in a degree of fixed rotation. In clinical practice we find that 'transverse pressures' work well to undo this. These are pressures with the thumbs, sideways against the small knobs of the back. They restore some of the lost rotation, causing an immediate reduction in pain. Pressures to the ribs where they key into the sides of the twisted spine also help. Again, as an overall approach, yoga is invaluable (see section on Yoga, Chapter 7).

WHAT IS VERTEBRAL STENOSIS?

Stenosis is a cramped cord in the spinal canal. It is described in Chapter 4 (see 'Do I Need an Operation?') as a complication of surgical intervention. But you can also be born with stenosis or you may acquire it through degenerative changes, when the internal bore of the spinal canal silts up with bone and tissue, like scale inside a kettle.

Whatever the cause, the spinal cord and nerves hanging down inside the canal are subjected to a very tight fit. The cramped conditions inside reduce the margin in which the highly sensitive neural matter can swing around and this leads to trouble. Although nothing seems amiss while you are inactive, as soon as you try walking, particularly uphill, it is a different story.

Normally, during the act of walking, the demand for action invokes an immediate response in the nerves activating the muscles of the legs. The nerves within the canal engorge themselves with blood in order to carry out their role. But if conditions are too cramped for the nerves to swell, the nerves themselves suffer blood starvation. This gives rise to diffuse cramping pains in one or both legs.

The pain is only ever evident while walking, be it on the flat or up steps or a slope. It can be distinguished from the similar cramping from vascular disease (with which it is often confused) because the pain intensifies over increasingly short distances, after you have rested to relieve it. In severe cases it may be necessary to squat to gain relief, since this broadens the internal dimensions of the canal and allows more blood to pass through to the nerves.

Many people have a narrower than usual spinal canal but never experience stenosis symptoms until some other development further reduces its dimensions. In such cases these space-occupying lesions – most commonly disc bulges or arthritic facet changes – make a tight fit even tighter.

With degenerative arthritis, there is proliferative bone growth and thickened soft tissues. These deposit themselves in and around all the joints and hinges of the spine and as a lumpy lining inside the canal.

A facet joint is most readily affected by this process. Stenosis here accounts for the picture of pain in one leg only. It is the result of silting up of a lateral exit canal (the intervertebral foramen) with bone and thickened tissue around the joint margins occluding the canal. It creates a physical stricture around the spinal nerve root which the nerve struggles to get past.

Often the degeneration of the facet is unobtrusive, with little evidence of backache along the way. It may take years for the characteristic cramping leg pain to come on. In these cases, the back degeneration was 'cold' rather than 'hot'; although there may have been a grumbling backache over the years, it was patchy and nothing like the bother of the more recent leg pain.

There can be an added complication. If the fuzzing up of the neural canal is accompanied by a degree of spondylolisthesis (or forward slip of a vertebra off the one below), the symptoms of vertebral stenosis can be even more marked.

The presence of spondylolisthesis creates a step in the inner tube of the spinal canal which produces a collar of constriction on the cord. In slipping out of place, the vertebra also makes a bony notch in the diameter of the intervertebral foramen which partially occludes the hole through which the spinal nerve must pass. Both anomalies can give rise to symptoms of stenosis. Furthermore, with spondylolisthesis, the ever-present possibility of increasing slippage of the upper vertebra results in increased wear and tear, which accelerates the other process. Arthritis on the rampage! The central canal and/or the intervertebral foramen are occluded even more.

Deterioration is often insidious and the most trivial of incidents can be the final straw – ricking the back getting out of the car or tripping on a step – and the neural canals become even more congested by local inflammation and swelling. It is cases like these which support my view on the mixed value of x-rays. There are those which almost defy the radiologist's powers of description because the pictures look so bleak. Yet, frequently, these are the people who barely knew they had a problem before the recent incident took place. This bodes well for their prognosis, though, despite the

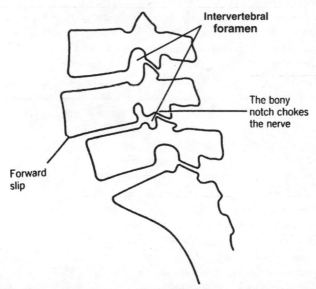

Figure 3.19 Spondylolisthesis can create a bony notch and occlude the foramen where the spinal nerve passes out of the spine.

appalling x-rays. And with appropriate treatment it may not be long before their ravaged backs are working as well and as painlessly as they ever did.

As with all problem back cases, the critical factor is the degree of internal inflammation and engorgement and whether, with my hands, I can cause this to subside without adding to the general hubbub. Manual therapy works well, especially if it is matched with tummy strengthening. But, even if we cannot shrink the soft-tissue build-up around the nerve root and the back does go to surgery, the post-operative result is much enhanced by pre-operative manual techniques to minimise the congestion and maximise tummy support.

WHAT WILL X-RAYS DO?

X-rays are important to exclude the presence of fractures, rheumatoid arthritis and tumours. They also tell us something about disc height, which is significant, but nothing beyond that. X-rays take *still* pictures of bones, but bones do not usually cause pain. It is the *joints*, those junctions of bone, held together by soft tissues, which cause the trouble. It is like taking a photograph of a door hinge. You cannot tell from the picture whether the hinge works or not. Of course, if there are lumps of rust hanging off it, you might fairly safely assume that things won't be running too smoothly – but then again, they might be.

There are thousands of instances of dreadful back pain where nothing shows up on X-ray, just as there are dreadful X-rays with never a day of pain. X-rays can and do pinpoint trouble sites by showing loss of disc height, which is the forerunner to most spinal ailments. They can also reveal if neuro-central joints and facet joints are moth-eaten and irregular at their margins which indicates instability (past or present) of that part of the segment. But even so, experience often shows that the level that looks bad may not be causing the trouble.

However, the presence of a problem joint on X-ray may not be entirely divorced from a pain felt elsewhere. The obvious-looking X-ray changes of gnarled and knobbly joints are rather like white ashes left after a fire. In many instances, however, the fire went out long ago; the 'activity' has died and the ashes are cold. The joint has gone through its agonies and is now quiescent. But as always, the legacy of former inflammation is dysfunction of the joint. This, in turn, throws extra strain on to the nearest joint, or the nearest but one.

This phenomenon also accounts for the classic criss-cross siting of trouble, back and forth across the spine, up and down its entire length. As lack of mobility of a facet on one side makes its effects felt, it translates strain diagonally across to the other side. This is more common in the neck than in the low back and accounts for the confusing picture of the 'pain everywhere' syndrome.

X-rays might show a joint on the right to be below par, but the poor joint up a level on the other side may be taking all the strain because the one below is not working properly. Although there may be pain, signs of strain may be too early to show on X-ray: bony changes often come on much later, long after functional performance has gone awry. X-rays tell us nothing about poor function, which, after all, is the reason for pain. 'Stiffness' does not show up on pictures.

Furthermore, soft-tissue structures are not 'radio-opaque'. Regardless of their state of health, they cannot be seen on X-ray, and therefore cannot be shown as troublesome. This includes the discs, which everybody gets so excited about. Bulges cannot be seen. Remember, the only thing we can deduce about a disc from an X-ray is its height. We certainly cannot see if it is bulging and pressing on or pinching a nerve. Mind you, a narrow disc in itself is reason to sit up and take note (see Chapter 2 'Do I Have a Stiff Spinal Segment?').

It would be an enormous help if there was such a tool as an X-ray video in use, to see segmental performance in action. It would then be a simple job to diagnose, as it moves, which segment of the spine is not moving properly, and whether the front or back compartment is primarily at fault (or both). As it stands at the moment, the only fail-safe way is to actually *feel* the spine as it moves.

If a surgeon is considering operating, he may do a myelogram or a radiculogram beforehand although, these days, both are largely outdated. Both involve injecting a radio-opaque dye into the internal canal space, waiting until it trickles around all the discs and nerve roots, and then X-raying the result. If there is abnormal bulging contour of a disc, which could conceivably be causing pressure damage, the surgeon would feel justified in removing that disc. But apart from that, X-rays are not much use at all. My clinic is piled high with people's abandoned X-rays which I have given but a cursory glance.

In recent times, myelography has been almost completely superceded by MRI (magnetic resonance imaging). These pictures give much more accurate, almost 3-D clarity images of the goings on inside a spine, and they have brought with them a great leap forward in spinal diagnostics.

4

A Choice of Treatments

Before I start talking about my favourite subject – treating spines with manual mobilisation – I want to give you a rundown on all the other treatment choices available.

In your quest for a cure I know most of you will have tried everything. Everybody has their very special person they swear by, or helpful piece of advice. Yet if you were to take up any of their suggestions, one might be invaluable, while another as helpful as fanning with a straw hat. The variety of 'cures' is limitless and eventually most of you will be wearily sceptical of listening to anything new.

The very fact there is such a variety of alternatives in spinal treatments points an incriminating finger to us in the medical profession. We have not come up with the one fail-safe way of fixing backs.

WHAT WILL TRACTION DO?

Traction is 'the rack'. It consists of a harness around the chest, and another around the hips attached to a variable weight. The patient lies relaxed on the back and the weight pulls or, rather, eases the spinal segments apart. In the absence of more localised and specific treatment techniques, traction can be the treatment of choice.

However, traction is a cumbersome arrangement, especially if it means traipsing into a hospital's outpatient department to avail yourself of its cures. It simply pulls all the vertebrae apart and you can do almost the same thing yourself using a BackBlock at home (see page 71).

Even so, traction does have its uses. I tend to use it rather as a fall-back technique to resort to if my continual handling of a problem joint in the course of treatment has made it sore. This is a common phenomenon and is referred to as treatment soreness (see 'Can Treatment Make Me Worse?' later in this chapter). Here, traction applied as a gentle, mechanical pull-and-release is helpful in dispersing bruising while still allowing the process of releasing the segments to take place. It is an effective, indirect way of

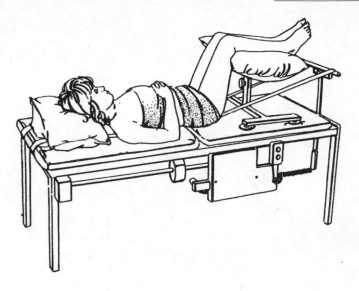

Figure 4.1 Low lumbar traction.

keeping things moving.

Traction is also useful in treating a severely swollen joint, which occurs when it is acutely inflamed. When a joint is literally too painful to be touched, it becomes locked in swollen rigidity. Movement causes pain but paradoxically, because it cannot be moved, it becomes more painful. The lack of movement makes the circulation in and out of the area slow down and the tissues become further engorged. The joints of the spinal segment will be tense and painful.

Normal to-and-fro movement of a healthy, functioning spinal segment acts like a pump by shunting blood in and out. It greatly boosts joint circulation. Without that movement, the blood-flow becomes sluggish and more swelling collects.

In this instance, extremely gentle, rhythmic, oscillatory traction (2–3 kilo pull or less) will encourage the joint to work normally again. The gentle pull and release of the traction for a brief period probably sets up a temporary artificial pump which establishes a better filling-and-emptying blood-flow through the soft tissues of the joint, which persists even after the traction has finished.

Static traction, which is a continuous distractive pull, can also be used to decongest a severely swollen joint. Here again, the weight of the pull is minimal. The effects, in this instance, are derived from the distraction of the two opposing bony surfaces. The sustained reduction of pressure within the joint for a short period of time (five minutes) is sufficient to allow the tissues time to drain themselves of their stagnant collection of used blood, whereafter new blood can be pumped in and dynamic circulation restored.

We physios run into trouble when we give a patient too heavy or too long a pull. It is then possible that pulling the joint apart can achieve the converse of what we are trying to do. The joint becomes engorged and bloated by the pooling of blood in the joint's soft tissues. If this happens, it is possible to feel much worse when the traction is released. There is then no other option but for the patient to go straight back onto the traction table again and for an hour or so, to have the weight of pull gradually reduced. We have all done this to someone at least once in our working life and, I can tell you, they cannot get out of there quickly enough. It is very bad management and most unfortunate.

Traction of a very different kilo pull (over 40 kilos) is very useful in treating a non-painful, chronically stiff back with advanced degenerative change present at every level. In such cases, the physio has to call up every technique in the book to get some movement in that stiff, prematurely aged back. Here, traction will be used in combination with vigorous manual mobilisation, treading on the spine – indeed, dancing on the spine (with the patient lying on the floor and the therapist hanging onto the treatment couch for stability) – and an elaborate variety of stretching exercises (including the BackBlock – see below) to be done at home between each treatment session. As the years have gone by, I have used traction less and the BackBlock more.

I am frequently asked whether hanging from a doorway does any good. It does. The only problem is that you have such a hard job holding on it is barely relaxed enough to be useful. Many patients feel it is exactly what their back needs, however, and I am totally in accord with them since I believe so in intuition. The fact is, this *may* help, but a BackBlock is infinitely better. (And so much more peaceful! You just lie there and gravity does everything.)

The last thing to say about traction concerns the 'Backswing' frames which snap around your ankles and allow you to hang upside down, relaxed and floppy, so that your vertebrae pull apart. The benefit you gain is directly proportional to the degree of relaxation. In general, Backswings are moderately effective, but their disadvantage is that maximum pull happens where there is minimal curve of the spine, which means at mid

The direction of the distractive force of traction

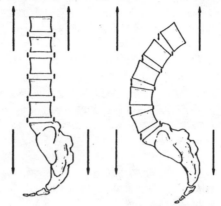

The direction of the distractive force of traction

Figure 4.2 If the spine is subject to a distractive force while it is curved, there is an unequal pull across partially opened joints.

to upper lumbar level. If you have a high lumbar problem, this is excellent, but most problems are lower down and barely benefit from this sort of pull.

USING A BACKBLOCK

But there is another way of getting the low vertebral segments to separate, which is a whole lot easier and more accurate than hanging upside down, not to mention cheaper. This employs the use of a BackBlock, a humble device based upon Iyengar Yoga. To me, a BackBlock is living proof of the dictum, 'simple is genius'. Who would have thought that something so unpretentious as a chunk of wood could be more helpful than just about anything else for an ailing spine? (See ordering details on page 202.)

Because our spine carries itself upright, over time the lower end telescopes into itself. If you imagine a vertical concertina which sinks and springs under the effects of gravity with every move the spine makes, it is not then hard to imagine the lower spinal segments compressing as we go about life. This is a fundamental truism of the human body. With the vertical compression of the column, the bricks at the bottom of the stack jam together because of all the superincumbent weight. Everything is pressed together as if the base of the spine were caught in a vice. Opposing bony surfaces of neighbouring vertebrae approximate, the discs flatten and fluid is squeezed out. More irreversibly, the binding soft tissues pucker as the spine shortens and becomes impacted, brittle and unresilient.

The business of sitting potentiates all this. The added compression bunches up the base of the spine even more. And remember, Westerners sit all the time – driving, eating, reading, writing, telephoning, sewing, typing, using a computer, watching television. Like a concertina where one end cannot be pulled out, the bottom end of our spines never gets a chance to drop down and disengage. Most of us are walking around with permanently jammed lower backs.

But there is another set of factors which predisposes us to trouble – and it's all to do with doing everything bent over. Our activity mode is always crumpled. As we concentrate our gaze over the task at hand, we curl forward. Whether we are using a computer, threading a needle or shearing sheep, we hunch over to focus our interest over a fairly small field of vision.

This predominance of one-way activity has long-term effects; we develop a stoop. Even if it isn't an obvious stoop, as a dynamic phenomenon, we lose the ability to go back the other way; to arch backwards. This permanent state of imbalance, superimposed on the impacted brittleness of our lower spine, means trouble is just beneath the surface. It is easy to hurt and, sooner or later, we invariably develop spinal pain.

This is where the BackBlock comes in. It undoes both sets of problems. It is an oblong piece of wood about half the thickness of a shoe box which you drape yourself over, backwards. This is the way to do it.

Begin by lying on your back on the floor. With your knees bent, lift up your pelvis and slide the Block under your bottom. It should fit quite comfortably under the sacrum, that hard flat bone at the base of the spine with the two dimples either side. From here, one at a time, allow both legs to straighten out along the floor and relax. Try to keep both heels together, although your feet will fall out. You must completely let go, so you feel a sensation of agreeable discomfort, a pulling-out feeling in the lower back and across the front of both hips. Don't be alarmed if you feel uneasy, even the familiar pain you have long complained of. That sweet pain will always be associated with a sense of release. It goes right to the nub of things and usually causes a specific local discomfort, deep inside, right where you know something is wrong.

The action of lying backwards passively over the Block, gently opens out the lower back, just like pulling out a concertina. Of all the myriad movements you have performed in your life, you have probably never done this. And it is remarkable that all you do is lie there while gravity does all the work. It separates the jammed lower vertebrae *and* takes you out of your habitual stoop. It is a brilliant combination, and really so simple.

Of course you can do similar backward arching in the prone lying position as shown in Figure 6.7.4, and standing as shown in Figure 6.7.5, Chapter 6. But, in both these procedures, although you get the benefit of the backward arch, you fail to get the traction or pulling apart of the lower vertebrae. Indeed, you get the converse – greater impaction, particularly of the facets, which in some instances you do not want.

The BackBlock can be used in progressive stages. Use it first on its flattest side, so that your bottom rests only seven or so centimetres off the floor. Once you have mastered this for one-minute spates, progress to using it on its middle edge, running crosswise under your sacrum. This raises you about 12 centimetres off the floor. Again, do this for one-minute periods only. The next advance is to turn the Block, still on the same edge, length-wise under your sacrum. The narrow edge of the Block is approximately the same width as your sacrum, so it allows the two sacro-iliac joints, at either side of the sacrum, to join in the stretch. Eventually, very lax-jointed people can progress to using it up on end (see Figure 4.3.6). But this should not be entered into willy-nilly, and, again, should be done for only one minute.

Simple as the BackBlock sounds, it is often astonishingly uncomfortable to start with. Some people (even those without a back problem), cannot stay on the flattest edge for longer than a few seconds. (They, incidentally, have problems in store.) This quickly improves as one slides the Block out, returns to the floor and does knee-to-chest bounces and curl ups before trying again.

I have taken to supplying BackBlocks to all of my patients. I provide them complete with explanations for use and the precautions. BackBlocks, quite simply, make my job *so* much easier. And what's more, once my patients are hooked, their days of seeing me are numbered. Once they can actually get themselves out of pain by using the Block, they never look back.

You can achieve a similar result by lying over a thick telephone book, but unfortunately this arrangement cannot be progressed so easily. I ask people to use their BackBlock every day. (I use one myself every evening to un-crimp after the day's toil.)

The important rejoinder about the BackBlock is that curl-ups must *always* follow, and you cannot afford to lapse. The sequence is always: BackBlock, knee bounces until the spine feels comfortable again, and then curl-ups. The longer you lie on the Block, the more curl-ups you must do

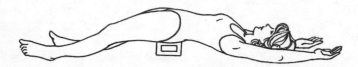

Figure 4.3.1 Lie on your back on the floor, knees bent, lift your bottom and slide the Block at its flattest, crosswise, under the hard, flat bone at the base of spine. Straighten one leg at a time out along the floor so that both legs are relaxed, heels together. Remain in this position for up to one minute (you may only manage a few seconds to start with).

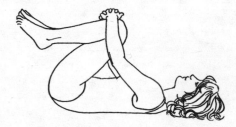

Figure 4.3.2 After coming off the Block, gather one knee up with the hands and bounce it gently towards the chest. Repeat with the other leg, then both together. Continue until the back feels comfortable again (15–30 seconds).

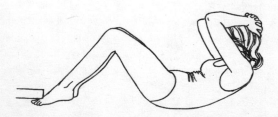

Figure 4.3.3 After coming off the Block and bouncing the knees, do up to 15 gentle sit-ups with the feet secured. The longer you lie on the Block, the more sit-ups you must do. If this is difficult, pull yourself up with you hands on your thighs, then return to the floor with your hands in front of your, instead of behind your head as shown. Curl up, roll down. Slowly! One segment at a time.

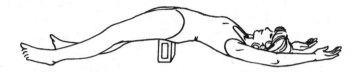

Figure 4.3.4 Progress by turning the Block onto the middle edge, crosswise, increasing the time as discomfort eases. Note: It often hurts to bend your knees and lift your weight off the block. Don't panic, everybody feels this.

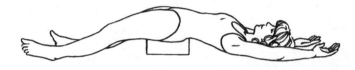

Figure 4.3.5 Progress by turning the Block, middle edge lengthwise, under the sacrum. As you find it easier to stay there, increase the duration up to 60 seconds. Do not stay longer in any one of the Block positions.

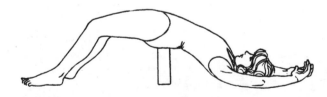

Figure 4.3.6 Only for the very fit. Stand Block upright on end. Progress the time you do this as before. It may take several months to progress through each successive phase.

(up to 15 for one minute). If you are stiff after using the Block (and this is quite common), you probably need to do more curl-ups and precede them with more knee bounces (as shown in Figures 6.9.1 and 6.9.2, Chapter 6) first with one leg at a time, then both knees together. Knee bounces are appeasing and allow the curl-ups to be done more easily.

SHOULD I NOT REST IN BED?

Bed rest is really cheating. The rationale is straightforward enough. If you can't be sure what the matter is, or what else to do, then bed rest will do no harm. Meanwhile, let's hope that whatever is wrong goes away in the meantime.

If the problem is lack of joint mobility – the most common back problem – then bed rest is about the last thing it needs – that is, if you are hoping to cure yourself. It simply allows the joint to get stiffer and the root cause to grow more intractable.

Although it is true that a brief spell horizontal may ease acute symptoms, the problem of poor segmental function will not be dealt with. By remaining untreated, it will sit there ready to complain again at the first opportunity, as soon as it is provoked by another awkward movement.

However, there are some instances where bed rest is ideal. When a spinal segment is so irritable that even the slightest movement brings on unbearable pain, physical treatment – that is, passively mobilising the segment – will only make matters worse. It is better to rest completely until the dust settles. This even means using bedpans instead of going to the lavatory, so that acute inflammation can die down.

Your bed must be firm; you must lie completely flat with only one pillow – never in a half-sitting position bolstered by cushions. In bed, you may move around as much as you like. All movements help, especially serpentine, wriggling ones where the segments have to disengage to move the body's bulk.

Bed rest helps with acutely inflamed conditions, whether of the disc or facets. If surgery to the disc is indicated but you are not keen, then the only way to relieve the pressure inside the back is to rest. By not imposing weight on the segement, you will buy time for the swelling to drain away so that all engorged structures can shrink. This may mean spending several weeks horizontal.

I believe a good deal of improvement in these cases is brought about by the settling of local inflammation which has added to the general hullaballoo inside the back. Remember, it is not simply the pressure from the disc which causes mischief; it is the whole 'metabolic climate' in there.

In fact, a good rest in bed does everything some good. It provides a much needed respite from your ordeal and temporarily removes you from the chaos of running a work-life while coping with intolerable pain. It allows you time to recoup energy, all your reserves having been depleted by the fight against pain. It allows time for the disc to shrink. It takes the spinal muscles out of action so they are more likely to relax, and it allows time for the general all-round swelling and inflammation in the area to disperse.

CAN MASSAGE HELP A PAINFUL BACK?

Massage is very agreeable, but only indirectly helps back pain. When a spinal segment is irritable, the overlying spinal muscles automatically go into involuntary 'protective muscle spasm'. This spasm in itself is uncomfortable, similar to a low-grade cramp. Its purpose is to temporarily splint the hurt joint so that it is not moved too much before it can take it. Sometimes the muscle spasm becomes extreme. This often happens because you are frightened and you add your own 'optional' muscle tenseness to the already-present automatic spasm. These muscles feel sore and tender to touch, but remember that they are only in spasm because a joint nearby is in trouble. By treating the muscle spasm with massage, you are treating the effect while ignoring the cause.

However, massage can help to 'soften' permanently over-tense muscles – in effect, working on the problem from the other end – with great therapeutic benefit. To explain how massage might work, though, I must briefly describe how muscles work and the differing roles of the two main muscle groups.

Muscles are composed of muscle fibres which clump together, side by side. The genius factor which makes muscles muscles and not some other soft tissue (such as tendon or ligament) is that muscles contract and shorten in length. Take the biceps, for example, which spans the elbow. At a given message from the brain, all the individual biceps fibres shorten themselves and thus magically bend the elbow. Because the shortening process always happens across a joint, the joint is made to bend. All muscles work this way and they all have their own joint. They act like pulleys working levers (the bones) and this is how the jointed skeleton moves us in its beautifully synchronised, streamlined way.

Broadly speaking, there are two basic muscle groups which interact to make us function with purpose. The first are the anti-gravity muscles, which are in action all the time. They keep the skeleton poised in an upright stance, making the background positional adjustments which set the stage for all the other whimsical phasic functions we might choose to do. The muscles in the anti-gravity group are larger with coarse, strong fibres – for example, the quadriceps, which brace the knees and prevent the legs buckling, and the gluteal muscles of the buttocks, which contract all the time and keep us from folding up at the hips. Another important group is the long, cord-like muscles of the spine which keep the torso from slumping forward.

Smaller, more delicate 'phasic' muscles perform all those other transient, elective motions that make up the living person, be it bringing a spoon to the mouth, smiling or simply tapping the foot to music.

The important fact is that the first group is on duty all the time – unlike the muscles of the second group, which come into play to make a fleeting appearance and then withdraw. For example, you might be roused to smile broadly. But your head is already in position, sitting up in the middle of your shoulders as a matter of course, because the muscles in the back of the neck are keeping it there. You do not have to exert any will over them, even though you might over the muscles that make you smile.

Anti-gravity muscles therefore have a laborious job. They operate by keeping up a monotonous state of low-grade contraction, quite unlike the phasic ones, which burst into a flurry of activity and then, when it is all over, settle back and relax.

The job of the anti-gravity muscles is made even more laborious if the postural alignment of the skeleton is so bad they must work overtime simply to keep the skeleton upright and poised for action. Anti-gravity muscles get sore. Furthermore, their 'overwork' is very taxing and, eventually, they lose the ability to relax, even after their role is no longer required.

This sustained, heightened contraction of the muscles is known as 'residually raised tone' or 'chronic muscle spasm'. If spasm is particularly relentless, some of the muscle fibres change in nature, losing their original qualities of contractability. They develop hard, tender cords, the old-fashioned name for which is 'fibrositis'. This is not a common cause of low backache; it is more usually a problem across the base of the neck and the back of the shoulders and is the result of the head being carried too far forward, in front of the line of gravity. The overworked trapezius muscle is always trying to pull the head back, like horse's reins, in line with the rest of the spine, and failing.

Massaging fibrositis helps break down the hard lumps and makes the tissues softer. This makes the muscles more comfortable, but permanent relief is only possible by loosening the joints of the neck and thorax and establishing a better posture so that *strain* disappears. Incidentally, the BackBlock under the upper back realigns the spine and takes away the typical strain of 'poker' neck. Placed flat and lengthwise, level with the top of the shoulders, it prises the spine straight and brings the neck back into line. It creates an absolutely marvellous sensation as it stretches everything out. At the same time, massage can break down the knots.

Another ideal application for massage is to promote relaxation. It is true that, in the presence of chronic back pain, lack of relaxation – that is tension – will increase pain (see 'Does Tension Make My Back Worse?' Chapter 8). Therefore, generalised body massage can bring about an all-round beatific state; something which is surely desirable. In this case, the massage can be gentle or hard, whichever proves the more relaxing.

WHAT WILL PILLS DO?

There are three groups of tablets which help you cope with pain, but do not expect too much from the pill-bottle. With a simple back problem that is unrelated to disease, no tablet will get rid of the underlying function fault, which is invariably the cause of the pain.

Pain-killers or Analgesics

Provided that you are undergoing physical treatment to undo the mechanical problem, there is no harm in making yourself a little more comfortable for the duration. Pain-killers are useful to knock the peak off the pain, especially if that pain has been temporarily increased by the treatment itself.

So far as choice of drugs is concerned, there is one golden rule: always listen to your doctor and follow prescribed dosages. This may be stating the obvious with prescription-only drugs such as codeine, but the rule applies with equal force to ordinary over-the-counter drugs such as aspirin or paracetamol.

Muscle Relaxants

As a natural automatic reflex, when a joint or disc is causing trouble, the overlying back muscles go into protective muscle spasm to protect that segment from further assault. These muscles are the caretakers of the joint, though usually, after a relatively brief period of time, once the muscles perceive the joint is moving slightly without causing pain, the muscle spasm fades. If you are in a heightened anxiety state, or if the trauma sustained by the segment is fairly severe, the muscle spasm remains intense and intractable. The sooner muscle spasm is eliminated, the better. It aggravates the hurt joint to have it bunched together by the overlying muscle spasm. Furthermore, treatment for the actual joint is held up while the muscle spasm is dealt with by the drugs. Muscle in spasm is also painful in its own right and is another source of pain.

Muscle relaxants help ease muscle spasm. They make the muscle caretakers sleepy and less vigilant. By reducing their hold, they allow the segment to make its first, tentative movements again. The pain-free movement shows the muscles that the cause for alarm has passed and their over-energetic attendance is no longer required.

Anti-inflammatory Drugs

Any joint that is not working properly is by nature 'inflamed'. The degree of inflammation varies, but by and large the pain increases as the degree of inflammation increases. Anti-inflammatory drugs act directly on inflammation to quell it. They also act to minimise the pain of treatment soreness when therapy has been aggressive and lengthy to undo the joint stiffness.

There are a number of anti-inflammatory drugs prescribed for back pain. Some, such as aspirin and indomethacin, have analgesic properties as well. Most, if not all, anti-inflammatory drugs have some side-effects. If you experience these, even at low dosage, you should try another compound. Typical side-effects include stomach pains, diarrhoea, nausea, dizziness and headaches. High blood pressure and pregnancy do not mix well with certain anti-inflammatory agents. You should never indiscriminately swallow medication on your own initiative; closely follow your doctor's orders. Also, remember never to commence or cease taking medication during a course of treatment because this will give an unrealistic reading on the progress of treatment.

SHOULD I HAVE SPINAL INJECTIONS?

In cases of severe back or leg pain which is aggravated by physical treatment and not responding to bed rest or tablets, it is often useful to inject a local dose of cortico-steroid (a powerful anti-inflammatory agent) right inside the working spinal joint to counteract the inflammation directly.

The spinal cord is the soft, squashy bundle of nerve pathways running down the inside of the spinal column from the base of the brain. Spinal nerves branch off all the way down the cord to leave the spine at each intervertebral level. The cord and its branches float in fluid inside a loose sack, the sack having continuous 'sleeves' covering the nerves until they are clear of the bony channels through which they leave the spine. This membranous sack is called the 'dura'.

An epidural injection squirts local anaesthetic and cortisone inside the spinal column, stopping short of the sack, in effect bathing the dura in this local medication. It is effective in quelling the inflammation of the nervous tissue and the sack (or sheath), thus reducing the pain. It may only take effect after making the pain worse for a day or two.

There is a branch of manipulative medicine which believes in the use of 'sclerosant' or 'sclerosin' injections. These are a sugar compound which, by irritating the soft tissues after injection, are said to cause scar tissue formation, which binds up a loose and over-wobbly joint and reduces symptoms caused by the irritable joint. Some practitioners appear to use sclerosants on all types of back problems – loose joints and stiff joints alike – and claim it helps everyone. I can't see how myself. It may be a placebo, or even have a counter-irritation effect whereby an 'old' pain is temporarily replaced by a 'new' one of a slightly different nature, thence permanently blocking the old pain pathway.

I do not know if these injections work; or, if they do work, why they work.

DO I NEED AN OPERATION?

A surgical operation on the spine may help in circumstances where there is unbearable pain (particularly leg pain) over a long period of time, unrelieved or made worse by manual treatment; where there are advanced and progressive neurological signs (such as loss of reflexes, numbness, pins and needles, loss of muscle power, and disturbance in sensation of the legs and/or saddle area with difficulty in passing urine).

There are two main operations for a bad back.

One is the *laminectomy*. This involves removing an irreversibly swollen disc and some of the nearby bone, by picking away at the bony canal through which the nerve travels on its way to the outside of the spine. This operation is not as drastic as it might seem; it does not weaken the spine's mechanical strength. It does, however, remove a vital shock absorber for the spine, leaving the segments to make virtual bone-to-bone contact. This also throws a greater weight-bearing load on the bony articulations at the back of the spine (the facet joints).

The complications after laminectomy are often brought about by failure to get moving soon enough afterwards. The prime consideration, therefore, after the first 24 hours following surgery, and after all the bleeding has stopped, is to get the spine mobilised again. Movement, using the back normally, is not dangerous.

When inactivity accompanies a bleed into tissues, the blood is not shunted away by the normal pumping action of natural movement. Instead, it pools and stagnates until it becomes so thick and gelatinous, it starts to clog up the delicate spinal machinery. If inactivity persists, this goo eventually becomes scar tissue, or 'adhesions', which is simply non-specialised, living junk. Continued inactivity allows this useless material to really take hold. It gets in around the nerve root, which has just been surgically freed, and brings about the very symptoms you have just had surgery to rectify.

It is important to stress that you need not expect to have a permanently handicapped spine after a laminectomy. Although there is an impressive scar left behind, the intrinsic length of the back has in no way been impaired – unless the surgeon has not repaired the thoraco-lumbar fascia beside the spine. Once again, there is absolutely no need for you to creep about as if your back is going to break. Movement is the best thing to make you feel normal again.

The unfortunate and unwelcome recurrence of the same degree of back pain after surgery, or even more leg pain (sciatica), has led to many a sad shake of the head and furrowed brow. However, it leads me again to assume that the disc bulge *per se* was not the sole cause of symptoms in the first place. It points to the possibility of the facet joint being part of the original problem.

If leg pain worsens after surgery, it usually indicates an existing facet problem has been aggravated. This happens because, as soon as you are upright, the two opposing surfaces of the problem facet, formerly kept apart by the presence of the disc, become jammed together (see Figure 4.4). The sciatica then worsens.

However, as mentioned earlier, scar tissue may proliferate out of control after surgery, and this may worsen pain. The amount of scarring depends on both the delicacy of the operative procedure and the inherent tendency of some individuals to scar (keloid). Thick, white, matted tissue infiltrates around the cord and the nerve roots and can sometimes almost strangle the nerve.

The development of sciatic pain resulting from scar tissue formation is slower and more insidious – say, six weeks as the scar develops – than in the case of a jammed facet joint, when the pain is almost instantaneous as soon as you are upright.

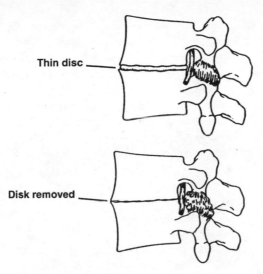

Thin disc

Disk removed

Figure 4.4 Grumbling facet joint trouble can be aggravated by joint-surface jamming after removal of a disc.

There is another explanation for persistent pain after surgery. One regularly sees in practice a laminectomy getting rid of more recent leg pain but not the original backache. In this instance, the disc is implied in the sciatica.

A common pattern with progressively troublesome backs is longstanding back pain which then develops into leg pain as well. This happens because the disc eventually starts to bulge, as a later phase in the sequence of breakdown, and the pressure this causes on the spinal nerve root causes leg pain. Although the surgery (a bulge-ectomy in effect) eases the discomfiture of the nerve, it does nothing to rectify the earlier symptoms caused by a dry and flattened disc making the spinal segment stiff. Surgery often relieves you of your secondary problem but does nothing to help the original one. In fact, it frequently makes it worse.

The second back operation is the spinal fusion. This is simply the surgical joining of one vertebra to another and is indicated when too much movement has developed at a vertebral level (segmental instability). That segment then becomes unstable, unable to be kept in place by strengthening the deep spinal 'intrinsic' muscles (see Chapter 6).

In the course of the same procedure, fusions are sometimes performed after a laminectomy. This pre-empts the disc removal bringing about a new sloppiness in the spine at the operated level. Previously, even though it caused problems, the disc had been a fairly competent spinal 'connector' holding its two segments together. Its robust width had kept its adjacent vertebrae well sprung apart and the spinal segment was therefore tightly functional. Removing a large part of the disc without fusing it afterwards often creates a man-made weak link in the spine.

Fusion may also be done to ease severe inflammation of a spinal segment. By obliterating all movement, the inflammation is allowed to settle.

The drawback with spinal fusion is that blocking movement at one level often leads to problems elsewhere. The lack of movement of the fused segment must be compensated for by over-movement somewhere else, at some level above or below the fused one. After several years, if not before, the compensating joint will show signs of irritation caused by excessive use, and this joint, too, will become a problem.

The other developmental problem of a spinal fusion is the insidious, progressive choking of the spinal nerves as they pass out of the spine, under the fused part. As we saw earlier, normal movement begets normal joints. Normal movement keeps a segment free, streamlined, efficient and uncongested. The reverse is true in a joint where movement has been artificially blocked.

For example, even in the absence of injury or disease, normal, healthy fingers that are kept immobile for a couple of days will puff up like a row of sausages. This happens simply because the pumping action of muscular activity has been stopped. As a result, the circulation slows and the digits fill up with fluid. (For this reason, incidentally, broken fingers these days are not splinted in plaster of Paris to allow the fracture to heal. They are simply strapped to a neighbouring healthy finger to keep the joint moving while the bone mends. This is because we now know that the acquired stiffness of the small finger joints is a much greater complication in the long term than the broken bone.)

During all operations there is a lot of surgical cutting of the tissues. Most 'bleeders' are tied off or zapped with the diathermy needle but blood and clear lymph fluid still ooze out, pooling and stagnating in the tissues. Because the joint has been splinted rigid by two large metal screws joining one vertebra to the next, the fluid is not dispersed by movement and then absorbed by the bloodstream. Instead, a backwater develops, a stasis of circulation around the fusion – the first step in the formation of 'adhesions'.

These adhesions may become so prolific that they severely clutter up the small channels through which the spinal nerves make their exit (the foraminae). The channels become choked and the nerve becomes physically hampered by this invasive undergrowth of living junk. Eventually the nerve can become completely bound up in scar tissue – so much so that it shrivels to a fraction of its normal size.

Another complication of fusion – and of laminectomy too, for that matter – is excessive new bone growth. This happens where the hard top layer of bone is bevelled away by a surgical chisel. Denuded of its hard top layer, new bone growth can proliferate. This, too, gets in the way of the nerves.

Heavy scarring or bone growth may not necessarily irritate the spinal nerves, because both are fairly benign. However, it may squeeze the nervous tissue to such a degree that it restricts its blood supply, and this means trouble.

In its normal, healthy state, the spinal cord and its branches, the spinal nerves have an abundant blood supply. This is so obvious that when exposed at surgery, they can be seen to pulsate with blood as each successive pulse-wave shunts through. A fine lacework of blood vessels climb all over a nerve, around and through the nervous tissue, keeping it supplied with generous quantities of good, clean, health-giving blood. The supply is quickly increased upon demand, with an escalation of muscle activity in the legs. When the blood supply is physically constricted by bony or fibrous entrapment, either within the spinal canal or the nerve root canal, the flow of blood that comes with each pulse beat is reduced to a trickle. When the area is exposed during an operation, the pulsation of blood coursing through the vascular network of the nerve is no longer obvious to the naked eye.

When extra work is demanded of the nerves – say, when climbing a hill or walking upstairs – the nerve itself suffers what is known as vascular embarrassment. You experience a particularly nasty pain in the leg which rapidly intensifies into a lead-like cramp as the walking continues. This syndrome is called spinal stenosis.

The pain in the leg is not dissimilar to the cramps caused by circulatory problems. The steeper the slope, the worse the pain. The only way to get relief is to stop walking. You feel an irresistible desire to sit down or squat to ease the pain. This curled position widens the diameter of the spinal canal (which is all fuzzed up with useless tissue clutter), thus allowing more room for a surging blood supply to pass through the nerve.

Stenosis can develop after surgery because of the proliferation of bone growth, which occurs when the top layer of bone is denuded. All bone is, in fact, soft tissue in a very hard form. Like all soft tissue, it weeps after trauma and then replaces itself in the healing process with bony 'callus'. The bone always produces more callus than needed, so, whether you have broken a leg or a surgeon has scraped away at bone with a chisel, excess bone will always develop at the site of activity. However, this can be disastrous if it develops inside the spine, because there is so little room – certainly not enough for any space-occupying matter along with the poor little nerve. The nerve gets squashed by this new growth – hence spinal stenosis occurs.

Developmental stenosis, when it occurs, is a very difficult state of affairs to rectify. It is counter-productive to go in again surgically since the same chain of events is likely to recur, with even more scar tissue formation next time.

Although many back operations are successful, they are essentially a last resort procedure. Manual therapy and restoration of trunk control should always be exhaustively tried before surgery is considered. In the case of spinal stenosis, mobilisation with the fingers does have a surprisingly effective role to play. The manual pressure may break down some of the fibrotic material by simply kneading it, but it is a long job. In the short term, it is much more likely that the pressure of touch brings about the relaxation of some of the muscles protecting the problem which, in turn, allows more blood to get through to feed the nerve.

SHOULD I TRY ACUPUNCTURE?

It must be said, there are cases where acupuncture succeeds when all else fails. I believe acupuncture is particularly useful in controlling back pain in cases where – even though the original problem has been cured – lingering muscle spasm persists, perhaps because the 'pain memory pathways' in the brain have been so well trodden that the messages continue to be passed, regardless of need.

Acupuncture in this instance seems to break the pain circuit. How it does this is not altogether clear. One suggestion is that inserting acupuncture needles into various parts of the body – not necessarily those feeling pain – may cause the release of pain-killing 'endorphines' (the body's natural opiates), thereby dampening sensitivity. Despite recent acknowledgements from conventional Western medicine that acupuncture does work, our understanding of it is still sketchy at best. However, I like it because it can do no harm, and, to me, its very subtlety is reason enough to sit up and take note.

WHAT IS MANIPULATION?

Manipulation is the therapeutic cracking of a joint with a quick thrust or tug. It is performed so quickly and deftly that it is impossible for the patient to prevent it happening.

In theory, it is sudden, manual over-pressure at the limit of a stiff joint's range, to open its surfaces. It is possible to learn the theory of manipulation but, without a natural aptitude, you will never do it with great finesse. Osteopaths and chiropractors pioneered the field of manipulative medicine and even today, on balance, probably do it with more flair and aplomb than the average physiotherapist.

Only relatively recently has manipulation been looked upon more favourably by conservative medicine. It was originally viewed as a dangerous fringe practice, which inevitably forced it further into the realms of crank medicine, with a lot of lay manipulators practising freely.

Manipulation is not dangerous if the patient is healthy. Stories of disasters (propagated by gleeful scaremongers) happen only when other medical conditions go undiagnosed beforehand, such as rheumatoid arthritis or bone tumours. Manipulation should not bear the blame. The skeleton, with its elastic ligaments holding its joints together, is pretty resilient. It is mandatory, however, that routine clinical investigations are carried out (by a doctor) beforehand to sift out conditions unsuitable for manipulation.

Manipulation usually produces a characteristic popping or cracking sound and many proposals have been put forward as to what makes the noise. I believe it is the suction caused by pulling apart the two joint surfaces. Two opposing surfaces usually hang together inside a joint capsule at a slight negative pressure, thus keeping close while lightly slipping past one another. When a joint becomes tight, the suction is greater and it is harder to pull the surfaces apart.

The academics say the popping noise is the formation and collapse of a gas bubble in a hundredth of a second . . . It is definitely not the breaking or tearing of adhesions nor the sound of bones being put back into place. Furthermore, there is no foundation whatever for claiming the sound is the sucking back and repositioning of a 'slipped' disc.

When a disc bulges, it is because the nucleus has ballooned off centre, causing the wall to swell out over a small focal area. The process never takes place instantly. It happens over a period of time as the disc's health deteriorates.

As we spend most of our time working, either bent over or sitting down, the lumbar spine compresses into a 'C' shape and the discs are all squashed out the back. After a time, the pressure causes the nucleii of the lowermost discs to start squirting through the inner layers of the disc's back retaining wall.

It is therefore unrealistic to expect that one yank on the poor disc can persuade its nucleus to relocate in the centre; it would be rather like trying to push toothpaste back into its tube, and then failing to screw the cap on. Even if it were possible to reposition the nucleus, it is asking too much to expect the split in the cartilage to then miraculously and instantaneously mend, when cartilage has no blood supply and takes months to regenerate.

The cracking sound is probably accompanied by an instantaneous breaking in the hold of the muscles on the joint. But, as comforting as that crack is, the sound alone has no therapeutic value. Healthier joints are easier to crack than unhealthy ones and the only relevance of the noise is that early on in treatment joints are less likely to crack, but, as their performance improves, they crack more. Manipulation is just as effective with or without a crack, but it takes some doing to convince a patient of that.

WHAT IS MOBILISATION?

The concept of manual joint mobilisation (Maitland Mobilisation) is the evolution of the life and work of Geoffrey D. Maitland, a physiotherapist from Adelaide, South Australia. He developed the concept from technical skill with his hands, combined with his knowledge of the other branches of manipulative medicine, which coalesced over the years into a carefully designed management of faulty joints. I am a non-purist disciple of Maitland. I have picked up a lot of his ideas and mixed them with a mash of my own.

So, we manual therapists are joint specialists. Joint performance is our speciality – not only spinal joints but also the peripheral joints, such as shoulders, knees, jaws and so on. Joints are a dynamic system; they are temperamental and prone to dysfunction, and they give the skeleton much more aggravation than the bones do!

It is always alarming to break a bone. But bones actually do quite well after being broken. Given time and a bit of splinting to hold the bone fragments together, they knit together in no time and actually end up stronger than they were originally.

However, the *joints* are often dreadfully mangled and pulled about by the same injury. Unfortunately, because they tolerate such a lot of shock with little outward signs of ill-effect, their lowered state of health and ongoing reduced performance can be easily overlooked.

Traditionally, stiff joints have never been seen as anything other than stiff joints; they have long escaped clinical scrutiny. Consequently, it is rarely realised that simple joint malfunction is capable of causing immense pain, either directly or indirectly.

The phenomenon of 'referred pain' can make it harder to trace general aches and pains because it often comes to light quite a long way away from the source. A diagnosis of 'fibrositis', 'muscle tear', 'ligament sprain', 'internal bruising', 'blood clot' and so on, can be made even though the real problem is a faulty functioning joint somewhere else.

In the process of treating a spine by manual mobilisation, we must first watch the spine do its major movements and note any deficiencies. We then use our hands to feel the individual mobility of each segment. This is done with the patient lying face down on the treatment couch – the spine spread out and relaxed, over a pillow, accessible to the investigative probing and pressing from the therapist's hands.

Areas of stiffness in the spine are immediately apparent. The block in spinal mobility feels like a plug of cement in a rubber hose. The vertebrae fail to slide away under pressure; they resist being moved and feel hard and unyielding on approach.

You, too, will be aware of something amiss when a stiff vertebra is pressured. There may be a local soreness, as if the bone itself is bruised, or perhaps a complete reproduction of the familiar back pain you have so long complained of. To all practical ends, it is not imperative to reproduce the exact pain; a comparable discomfort is proof enough that this is where the trouble is.

The pain may be reproduced by the problem vertebra being loathe to participate in one of its freedoms of movement – caused by a local shrinkage of the soft-tissues which wrap up the spine. For instance, it may be quite free to glide forwards and backwards on the vertebra below, but completely blocked and painfully resistant to swivelling on its axis. Conversely, it may be free to swivel but blocked to forwards/backwards gliding. These deficiencies in mobility constitute a fault of function and will be a source of pain, sometimes longstanding, as well as the source of other pains. It is important for a manual therapist to know this, and it is central to how manual therapy works.

The therapeutic part of the process follows. The therapist finds the rusty spinal segment with her thumbs and gently prises it free. This is done with gentle push-and-release pressures, usually with the thumbs, but perhaps with the heel of the hand, the knee, the elbow or even the heel of the foot.

Quite quickly, the vertebra begins to move again and participates as it

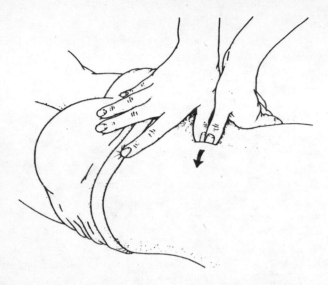

Figure 4.5.1 Mobilisation with the thumbs will loosen a stiff vertebra. It can be done in a transverse direction so that the vertebra swivels on its axis, or in a forward (and release) direction to make the vertebra freer to glide forward and back.

should in total spinal mobility. The length of time it takes to free a stiff segment depends on how long it has taken to get into such a state. It may take only one session if you developed the problem yesterday. Or, if you have had it for years; you may need intensive treatment for six weeks with follow-up booster sessions every six months for the rest of your life. It helps to do your own maintenance exercises (see Chapter 6), especially using a BackBlock to decompress the spine first. Then it is easier to reverse specific movement anomalies.

The key difference between manipulation and mobilisation is that mobilisation is geared to the state of the joint's soreness and debility. Treatment is geared to how much pushing the joint can take. As it becomes freer and less painful, the pressures can increase. Eventually the vertebra can be freely and painlessly pushed in all directions. Manipulation, on the other hand, pushes the joint instantly to its limits, regardless of its state of health.

The graduation of mobilising pressures varies from butterfly-light to extremely heavy-handed. In the case of the latter, lying the patient prone on the floor, and standing – even bouncing – on the spinal blockage will be the only way to get the spinal segment going again. On the other hand, very gentle pushing, pulling and gliding may be appropriate, even though you may feel that not enough is being done to make you better, especially if you are the type who believes everything has to be agony if it is going to work!

There are very specific reasons for using gentle techniques or hefty techniques. The longer I practise, the more I use both extremes. I frequently stand on backs.

SHOULD TREATMENT HURT?

Broadly speaking, treatment is designed to get rid of pain and, after that, to get rid of the dysfunction, usually stiffness, which by its presence has caused the pain.

Treatment to relieve pain is so gentle, it is comforting. You are simply having the joint persuasively coaxed into more and more movement. As movement returns, the severe pain that was present, even when you were doing nothing, soon disappears.

Then we arrive at the slightly more tricky stage of treatment where fine judgement is required of the therapist. The pain has become much more bearable, but, in order to continue improving the problem and treat the root cause, one has to start tackling the lack of joint mobility, too. In effect, the physiotherapist is juggling with both sides of the problem at once: reducing the residual inflammation, while at the same time starting to push and tug the joint to restore its original function, the lack of which initially caused the pain. This treatment in itself can hurt and cause new pain – treatment soreness. It should be easy to see why progress is sometimes a bit up and down!

In a way, by physically handling and stretching the joint, the physio-therapist is artificially irritating it – by gently provoking it so that the body's defences rally and send blood rushing to the site of the activity. A good physio will not overdo this forced inflammation. He or she should just stir things up enough to cause a little soreness, leaving a bruised feeling in the evening following treatment. When this subsides, the patient should notice a new freedom, and progressively less pain. (If you feel more than this you are being 'overdone', and you need to let your therapist know.)

When a back problem is more of a nuisance than painful, the spinal segment is usually just stiff and is hardly sensitive at all. At this stage, treatment is designed to get rid of the segmental stiffness. It is as hefty as the physiotherapist is strong. In my own clinic, two of us will sometimes get onto a patient's spine and he or she may be sore for days afterwards. (It should be a 'new', more superficial soreness, and nothing like the deep, gnawing ache of old.)

CAN I BE OVER-TREATED?

Treatment itself causes its own soreness and since this can mimic the original pain, it may be impossible to differentiate between the two. You may think that you are worse, or that you still need therapy because you still have pain.

It is common for a patient to be discharged from treatment still suffering some pain. But we may want to leave you alone and allow time to play its role in settling this man-made pain. You may return for treatment in six weeks, just to make sure there is nothing left of the original problem and that the newer temporary pain has gone.

At the other extreme, your physio may want to drag you back for treatment long after your pain has gone. Be assured that there is a good reason for this. If a segment is still lacking freedom, mobilising should continue until it is running smoothly in every direction.

We physios are very interested in what we call 'accessory movement' of joints. When any joint bends – say, for example, the elbow – it is not just a pure hinging action taking place between two bones. There is a lot of unseen shuffling, swivelling and gliding between the bones, as well as that obvious main movement.

The liberty to do this gives the joint a relaxed, floppy feel when it is handled by experienced hands. The joint feels empty and loose. Wonderful! It is healthy. When a joint starts to deteriorate, this invisible freedom is the first thing to go. The joint starts to feel tight and hard, and when it is professionally assessed, it is loath to go in some of its 'unusual' directions. If a joint is to be put absolutely right, then we must persevere with loosening it until full 'play' is back. The joint will then feel nice and empty again, like a loose bag of bones.

You might think we are making a lot of fuss about nothing; you can lift a cup to your mouth – what is the problem? However, if we do not fully mobilise that elbow, it will seize up again and you will be returning for more treatment sooner rather than later. The same applies with the joints of the back.

CAN TREATMENT MAKE ME WORSE?

In many ways, treatment is like scratching a scab to make it heal.

Because treatment provokes a reaction, it is possible in the short term to feel worse. However, your condition may actually be improving. As long as the function of the joint is becoming more normal, any pains, either new or old, will eventually disappear. The problem you must grapple with at this stage is your lack of confidence in the treatment (and the person administering it).

If you have not been previously warned about treatment soreness or were inadequately comforted at the time, you may drop out from treatment, feeling that the treatment has made you worse. Time would have told you that you are better but, sadly, some patients are not prepared to wait and see.

To sum up this chapter, there are a variety of treatments and procedures available for the back sufferer, but the most effective is joint mobilisation (followed by muscle re-education to enhance trunk control). I belive all the others are ancillary to this.

Whatever form of treatment you undergo, make sure your therapist is fully qualified. Never consult an acupuncturist, for example, without doing a little checking first on his qualifications, experience and reputation.

By now you should know enough about my own technique – mobilisation – to ascertain from any prospective physio how he or she plans to proceed. Don't drive her mad with questions on the telephone, though, because that will only waste time and get her back up. However, with treatment, you should know exactly what to expect and what is unacceptable practice.

5 Benefits of Mobilisation and Manipulation

Mobilisation of a joint is a subtle business. Unlike manipulation, there is no drama, no flamboyant thrusts and flourishes. And although the benefits take longer to be realised, the process is kinder to the joints and the effects are longer lasting.

Unlike osteopaths or chiropractors, physiotherapists do not manipulate every back that walks through the door. We manipulate only when there are specific indications to do so. We believe living tissue responds better to persuasive joint-stretching techniques to free it progressively over time, rather than one sudden jerk to break a joint free in a moment.

WHAT WILL MOBILISATION ACHIEVE?

A joint will be painful for one of two reasons. If you have been suffering for a while, the tissues around the joint will be stiff, making it hurt to bend through the stiffness. With an acute episode, a joint may be painful because it is swollen, but otherwise not the slightest bit stiff. The first is a chronic state and the second the acute state after recent trauma.

There is a third reason as well – a combination of the two – an acute injury superimposed on a chronic condition (the most common state of all). Chronically stiff joints are much more susceptible to repeat trauma, simply because they cannot roll with the punches.

All three types of disability are helped by mobilisation. Getting rid of the *stiffness* of a chronic condition is easy to understand. The same principle applies to a rusty hinge on a door: work it back and forth and you will knock off some of the corrosive scale so that it moves more freely.

Getting rid of *pain* in a chronic condition, when the joint has become tight, is more complicated. The joint is painful because movement stretches and tugs the stiff structures and, because it is unyielding, the stretch causes pain.

In the spine, it is easy enough to get rid of the pain by simply making the disc wall, the facet capsules and the surrounding soft tissues more elastic so

94

they accept stretch more readily. Persuasive mobilising – the manual stretching of a joint – will achieve this fairly quickly, though it may cause pain, albeit a 'sweet' pain, in the process.

With recent trauma, a virgin joint can be yanked about so it swells and becomes tensely painful. Equally, an old joint that has been stiff for years can be provoked anew, causing more inflammation and swelling on top of the pre-existing stuff. In either case, gentle, rhythmic joint movement rids the joint of fluid and eases the pain.

Apart from the movement pumping the joint empty of swelling, the highbrow neurophysiological explanation for the reduction of pain is as follows: the new nerve messages describing the gentle movement, now being superimposed upon the joint, effectively block or dampen former incoming messages about pain.

The familiar automatic response of vigorously shaking the hand, having just smashed your thumb with a hammer, helps describe this phenomenon. It feels better if you shake it – just as if you wrench your knee, your instinctive reaction of waggling it back and forth makes it feel better. Although you don't know it, your brain is being bombarded with messages about gentle movement in preference to the messages about nasty pain. One message overrides the other.

Physiotherapists who manually mobilise a painful joint try to achieve a similar end. Treatment is just a professional waggle of the joint, but geared to what the joint can take.

Movement also has the wonderful advantage of pumping the swelling out of a joint so it can move more freely. Conversely, if it remains still, the joint will become more swollen. During activity, the muscles that contract and release around a joint squeeze blood and waste materials out of the tissues and back into the circulation. Hence the joint loses its puffiness. The less a joint moves, the less it empties and the more swollen and painful it becomes.

People are often surprised when I attempt mobilisation very early after injury. It seems to fly in the face of all previously held convictions about 'rest' after trauma. As a rule, the earlier you start moving, the better. Generally, people rest too much. If you don't move an ankle, for instance, for a week after the injury, it gets not only more painful but also more swollen. It then takes much longer (and is more painful) to get moving later on. This is because all the fluid pooling in the tissues is well on the way to becoming hard, gristly scar tissue. This means more physiotherapy, as all scarring must be broken down and softened before it can be absorbed by the bloodstream. If the scarring stays there, the joint will remain painful and it is unlikely to move freely again.

After early treatment, subsequent mobilising is much less sore. It is not uncommon for a patient to suspect that the therapist has stealthily switched to treating some other spinal level, because it feels so much better. Simple, uncomplicated movement lifts a lot of the pain, and this is the beginning of mobilising a stiff spinal segment.

Once the pain has been dealt with, if it is an old or chronic problem, then the matter of stiffness must be tackled. To render a joint problem free, that stiffness must be reversed, or the same pattern of inflammation will recur.

As the stiffness eases and the joint becomes more elastic, the pain lessens. Then the mobilisation pressures increase. This highlights again the fundamental difference between manipulation, which is always carried out at the same strength and speed, and mobilisation, which is carefully graded to the ability of the joint to take the force.

CAN I MANUALLY MOBILISE MY OWN SPINE?

Ideally, yes, but in practice it is difficult.

As simple as the concept of manual spinal mobilisation is, it is very difficult to do on oneself. Believe me, I have tried. It is almost impossible to get one's own fingers into a position to do anything useful and all you do is make it sore.

In treatment, after we have located the problem level, both by watching full spinal movement and by feeling the segmental movement, we then work that segment free. In so doing, we may even have to lean on it with our full body weight (using the thumbs, the heel of the hand, the elbow or the knee), or even stand and tread on the stiff patch. So, as you can see, it is fairly hard to duplicate the same action on yourself.

Of course, general spinal movements of forward/back bending, left/right sideways bending, and twisting left/right do rely on all the individual segments doing the same to bring about the overall action. So it is true that these general movements, done vigorously and fully to the end of range, help restore segmental mobility. But there is a tendency for the fitter, more mobile neighbouring segments to compensate, instead of the stiffer, inactive ones being roused.

For the best outcome, the individual problem vertebra has to be sought and sorted out by the therapist's thumbs, right at the site of the trouble. Once again, background mobility and increased separation of the spinal segments can be achieved by using a BackBlock. As a first measure, this

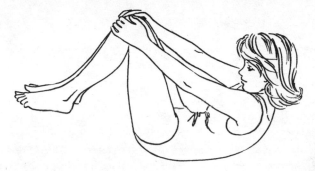

Figure 5.1 The best self-mobilisation technique is to roll the weight of the body back and forth over the problem link. Use small movements, almost like pivoting.

gives all the lumbar segments more room to move. This is particularly relevant if a vertebra is not only stiff but also twisted on its axis, like a screw-top lid of a jar wrongly screwed down. In this case, the tail of the vertebra may be swung across one way. From the 'outside' it feels out of alignment, but more importantly, it will be loath to go back *into* line. Only mobilising with thumbs will achieve this. It is like prising a champagne cork out of a bottle. Once again, the process will be greatly speeded up by separating the segments first with the BackBlock.

However, there is one especially good way of restoring forward/back segmental freedom, and that is rolling along the spine. This is done by lying on the floor on your back, legs held behind or on top of the knees with linked fingers, and gently rocking back and forth over the stiff patch. (It will feel slightly painful as you roll over it.) It is extremely effective and should be done for a few moments several times a day. Another version of this exercise, more localised to the lowermost lumbar levels, is rolling around the sacrum in a circular fashion. Start from the same position, holding the knees, and inscribe a wide circle in the air with your knees. This presses your low back into the carpet, as you visualise yourself tracing the triangular outline of the sacrum.

THE MA ROLLER

Another effective method of mobilising your spine – particularly the chain of facet joints running down either side – is using a Ma Roller. The Roller looks like a convoluted rolling pin; it is made from pinewood and has two large, rounded humps either side of a central hollow. (See ordering details on page 202.)

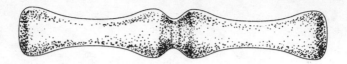

Figure 5.2 The Ma roller.

You use it by lying on your back on the carpet and rolling on it. Your knees should be bent to control the amount of weight on the roller and then you simply move up and down over it, a small section at a time. As you do this, the two humps pass over the bilateral chain of facets running down either side the line of the knobs you can see through the skin. These small back-and-forth movements break up the brittle immobility of the facets and pummel pliability into the tough capsular ligaments. Continue this action for a few seconds only. Too much can make you sore.

You may find you get better leverage and manoeuvrability if you support yourself on your elbows. You can then use the roller up under the rib cage where it is much more bony. It also helps to cradle your head in your hands.

Unfortunately, excellent as the Ma Roller is, some people are either too tender or too bony to have success with it. In its stead I have come to rely upon the lowly tennis ball. Not so lowly I suppose, because it must be new and top-quality, and therefore fully tensed. It is used in exactly the same way as the roller. Find the painful spot, lower your back down onto the ball, and then gently wriggle about on it. The stiff facet joint will be unable to move in concert with the rest as you roll over it, and you will feel its sweet, familiar pain. You may not necessarily sense its stiffness, but you will certainly sense pain. Roll back and forth over the ball for a minute, two or three times a week (more often will make you sore) and see how the pain fades.

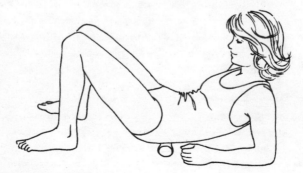

Figure 5.3 Ma Roller under lower back.

Many of my patients are addicted to their tennis ball and I have come to the conclusion that no family medical chest is complete without one. If self-treatment of a facet problem is to be taken seriously, this, in conjunction with the BackBlock, is the best means of self-mobilisation. Nearly as good as thumbs!

WHAT WILL MANIPULATION ACHIEVE?

Manipulation is particularly useful in unlocking an otherwise mobile healthy joint which, while it was not previously painful, has become jammed by an awkward movement.

Manual therapists also manipulate a degenerated joint when it is nearly better. Manipulation at this stage will get the spring back into the joint, thus speeding up the later stages of recovery. In the trade we call this 'clearing' the joint.

There is no doubt that the immediate feeling of release after a successful manipulation does bring about a sense of well-being. However, cracking like this is often too rough. Too many tissue fibres are broken, and although there is an initial sense of freedom, the relief quickly fades. You eventually become addicted to being yanked. Microscopic scarring forms around the joint which makes it tighter and tighter, so you feel that you need manipulating more and more frequently to keep yourself in the same free state.

As a manipulator myself, I know well the feel of a back which has been manipulated too often. The joints feel characteristically over-tough and rubbery and, even in the neck, they can be so hard to budge I feel I am wrestling a steer to the ground to get that tiny, elusive click. This is not a good way to go. Far better is protracted mobilisation (gently and perhaps for months), until the joints can be restored to their looser, more elastic state.

The other great problem with manipulative treatment, especially when done by lay manipulators, is that it is quite difficult to accurately localise the manipulation to the required spinal level. All manipulative techniques are done as a gross movement, using the rest of the patient's body for leverage. For this reason, it is very difficult to make the vertebral level go where you want it to go. Frequently there is a loud crack and everybody is very satisfied but, in reality, the healthy joint above has been treated and the real troublemaker has scraped by, untouched. This will not fix the problem.

A more satisfactory approach is to do a lot of preliminary mobilising with the thumbs (heel of the hand, elbow or heel of the foot) right on the spot to prise the vertebra free. Then, when it is moving more freely and one can get a bit more purchase, manipulate it.

Manipulation at the culmination of treatment of a problem joint is essential for its complete recovery. There is none of the adverse response described earlier because the joint, having been thoroughly worked over during several treatment sessions, is in a fitter state to accept more aggressive handling.

During the mobilisation process, the professional handling of the joint has brought the blood rushing to help it cope with the unexpected work load. Now, with the benefit of an improved blood supply, the tissues revert to a healthier state.

CAN MANIPULATION BE BAD FOR ME?

Manipulation is not dangerous with healthy people. However, it should never be done if the patient is pregnant or where there is rheumatoid arthritis, osteoporosis (where the bones become brittle) or bone cancer. Here it could be catastrophic.

That aside, joints should not be over-manipulated. It is easy to tell if you have had too much manipulation because your joints will have a rubbery, tight, spongy feel and will always be itching to be manipulated anew. The joint capsules become scarred and thickened by repeated forceful yanks which, in turn, cause more microscopic tearing and scarring of the tissue fibres. The scarring causes the joint to tighten up even more, so the force needed to gain movement next time is even greater. Scarring increases and the problem snowballs.

As a finale to a course of treatment, we often manipulate a joint just before final discharge. We do this to 'clear' the joint. This final demand ensures the joint is fully capable of moving freely and forestalls relapse due to incomplete treatment.

I know exactly what my patients like about these manual therapy techniques. They correspond closely, it seems, with what they instinctively feel their back needs. Surely, this is how medicine used to be, 'the laying on of hands' so sadly missing in today's impersonal, clinical world. The hands, in all their complex simplicity. The benefits are so clear-cut, they can hardly be overstated.

But, like most things in life, effective treatment of back pain is not just a one-sided affair. You, as a patient, must contribute largely to your own recovery. So far, I have outlined my role in easing a painful back. What follows now is how you can help yourself; something you should do progressively, more and more as treatment proceeds.

6 Exercises for a Back Problem

One of the most distressing aspects of a back problem is that sufferers see themselves as passive victims of pain. They feel unable to cope during an attack and equally unable to prevent a recurrence in the future.

However, you *can* help yourself. You can do one or two things right in the middle of an attack which will help to get rid of pain (these will be discussed later on). You can also do exercises that directly target the central problem, thus redressing the structural core anomalies that, by their very existence, have caused the trouble in the first place. This is what gives you a lasting cure.

Often, patients wonder why their back is bad when they are so active and play so much sport. But, the benefits of individual exercise and sporting activity are worlds apart. The value of sport is its capacity to rev up the system and put it into full flight, all in the name of fun. This has the hidden benefit of keeping the musculature toned up, of preventing muscle and ligament contracture and keeping the joints well oiled – in short, preventing the skeleton from getting out of shape. Ideally it prevents back problems starting in the first place.

But, the shortcoming of general sporting exercise is that it is not careful enough. It is hardly tailored to delicately undo the things which have gone wrong with a skeleton; more to the point, its blunderbuss effect, where joints, muscles and tendons are railroaded into action, often triggers dormant problems. Sport frequently fails to balance joint performance simply because it is not sufficiently balanced or controlled itself. Too often it is violent, with monotonous movement patterns subjecting the skeleton to fleeting new strains on top of pre-existing ones (see 'Sport And The Back' Chapter 7).

Sadly, most of us have skeletons with a patchy distribution of joints which are below par. Some are too tight while others are too loose, mostly from our lack of variety of activities *and* our resting postures; always in a chair watching television, hardly moving for hours at a stretch. It is then but a small step to 'do something' fairly minor which tips the balance. So often people complain that they hardly did anything to precipitate a particularly nasty bout of back pain. This causes frustration and a sense of hopelessness because you feel that if you can't even sneeze without disastrous consequences, then how are you to cope with the rest of life's rigours?

But, you see, you really had it coming to you! Your frame can be compared to a car where some bolts were rusty, some were not screwed up tight enough while others were over-tightened. All in all, an extremely creaky car. Its poor performance cannot be rectified by paying attention to just one bolt. Nor can it be rectified by taking the car on a hundred-mile drive – the equivalent of indiscriminate over-energetic exercising. The nuts and bolts of the skeleton can be equally out of whack.

If you are to spend a life as free as possible from aches and pains, it is important that the skeleton be completely balanced in all its physical work. For it to run harmoniously, there must be a balance of muscle play across all its working parts. But smooth-running joint performance can only happen if the joints are not stiff and if the muscles that control them are equally matched.

Each muscle group across a joint has an opposite number on the other side which provides the reciprocal movement. For example, the biceps bends the elbow and the triceps straightens it out again. The opposing group also performs the important, though less obvious, task of controlling the primary movement as it takes place. It does this by slowly relaxing and paying out its length so the primary movement is controlled, as it were, by the other side. The opposing muscle group keeps its tension on and only lets go at a delicately programmed rate, so the primary movement is smooth and purposeful, not jerky and uncoordinated.

It is important that all paired muscles are of equal strength and equal length. If a skeleton is bedevilled by joints with unequally matched partners, they will chafe. It doesn't do to have two masters of unequal ability controlling a joint. It leads to grumbling dissent; their threshold is lowered and they are more susceptible to injury.

Inequality of strength across a joint is easier to understand than the problems of length. If one group is stronger, it will powerfully pull a joint its own way, more easily than its partner can return it.

When it comes to stabilising a joint – as when bracing the back – both partners (the tummy and back muscles) have to contract statically to hold the joint (in this case the spine) firm to resist shock. If one group is holding more firmly than the other, it leads to trouble. It would be better if both were weak, rather than one weak and the other strong. The imbalance causes strain and shock to be tolerated poorly, whereas if both are weak, the resulting joint laxity helps the joint to ride out the storm with equanimity.

In the case of the back, muscle imbalance can affect several spinal levels. It sets the stage for any one of them breaking down. When the tummy is weak and the low back is in the clutch of permanent spasm, the row of spinal segments stacked on top of one another are much more susceptible to being ricked.

The stronger a muscle is, the more 'tone' it has. Tone is best described as the tension within a muscle when it is at rest, as if the muscle is in a permanent state of low-grade contraction. The greater the tone, the less extensible the muscle is. This means that, over a period of time, the muscle imperceptibly pulls in its length and becomes shorter. This is bad news for the joint underlying a strong muscle, not only because it spends its resting moments compressed under the non-relaxing muscle, but also because it is not as stretchy as a weaker muscle and can never let go and release to full stretch. Thus the joint never enjoys excursions up to the weaker muscle's end of range. When its turn comes to work, the weaker muscle is without the power to pull the joint against the resistance of the stronger group and it is harder for the joint to work one way.

Inequality of movement is therefore established. Over a period of time the stronger muscle adaptively shortens and the weaker one adaptively lengthens and a permanent contracture of the joint comes about.

The elbow is a good example of this. If a strong man spends more time bending his elbow rather than straightening it, his elbow will start to hang crookedly at his side, like an ape's, because he has lost the freedom to straighten it fully.

'Tennis elbow' is a condition caused by inequality in length of paired muscle groups. Because there are many more forehand shots in tennis than backhand, the flexor group on the inside of the forearm powerfully pull the wrist through with the racket. They get stronger than the extensor group on the back of the forearm which takes the wrist and racket back the other way, in the backhand shot. Because the punchy forehand slash is so powerful, the weaker extensor group on the back of the forearm is at a loss to exert proper control over the movement. They suffer a sudden jerk as they try to steady the wrist, the jerk tugging the muscle where it attaches to the bone at the outside of the elbow.

Furthermore, the strong forehand shot demands such total and instantaneous release of the opposing group, that even the shortest delay

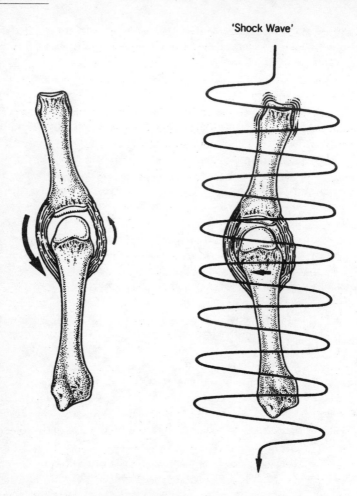

'Shock Wave'

Figure 6.1 Even at rest, a joint will suffer strain if held by a pair of muscles of unequal ability. If the joint is shocked, inadequate bracing will cause further damage.

results in the muscle being wrenched where it attaches to the bone on the outside of the elbow.

And because the flexor group is so strong, a backhand shot struggles to stretch it out to its full length. It cannot 'give' and pay out freely as the extensors contract to bring the racket through. While the feeble extensors are doing their best to pull the wrist back, the movement is suddenly pulled up short, in full flight, because the strong group has come to the end of its range. This jars the extensors again and causes a tug to ripple through the muscle, tweaking it where it is attached to the bone. This causes inflammation and pain at the tendon-to-bone junction. The familiar tennis elbow pain ensues.

This well-known example of how a joint can malfunction (sometimes producing arm-crippling pain) illustrates all too clearly how important the phenomenon is to all joints, not least the back. Muscles *must be of balanced ability* if joints are to work smoothly to co-ordinate the skeleton. The back is a good example because with so many of us, our tummies are weak. And this wreaks havoc.

It should now be clear why you should never concentrate on exercising one muscle group at the expense of others. The muscles at the front of the spine (the tummy muscles) and those behind (the back muscles), as well as those at the front of the hips and back of the thighs (the hamstrings), all have to be checked to see they are equally supple *and* equally strong.

Imbalance of the large skeletal muscle groups is a fundamental of human back trouble. It takes years to develop and will only come to light when you try to assume an anatomically perfect posture. Then it will be clear that some muscles are tight and cannot let you go, while others are weak and cannot get you there.

Stretching and strengthening exercises will make sure that basic good posture is yours.

WHAT EXERCISES SHOULD I DO?

Specific exercises may be necessary to restore parity to coupled muscle groups, but it is no use exercising indiscriminately.

If you are to take on the job of helping to treat your own back, you will not know what to stretch and what to strengthen until the basic posture types are understood. Exercises that are invaluable for one back may be disastrous for another.

But before any exercises start, the rationale of using a BackBlock must be explained because decompressing the spine, which is the same as pulling the segments apart, is the cornerstone of all spinal treatments.

Vertical compression is the root cause of most developmental spinal problems. What starts off as a benign flattening of the lower discs can become less and less reversible, until it leads to more serious problems of the disc-vertebra-disc compartment (at the front of the spine) or the facets (at the back of the spine) at the same level. Facet breakdown usually develops as a consequence of their bearing too much weight because the disc has become too thin. But it can also occur when the lumbar spine carries itself with too much lumbar hollow. Conversely, the disc-vertebra complex will suffer greater wear if the lumbar spine adopts too much of a stoop, making all the weight pass down through the neuro-central core and none through the facets.

In all these instances, using a BackBlock under the sacrum (and sometimes under the thoracic spine also) restores optimal lumbar posture, as well as the much soughtafter decompression of the spinal base. It is not so much an exercise as a procedure, aimed at redressing the fundamental flaws of the human skeleton's experience. Using the BackBlock for as little as a minute a day can make all the difference in making a spine work optimally again.

Having restored spinal alignment and started enticing fluid back into the discs to bolster shock absorption, the next step is to encourage better interplay between the muscles working the spine. This is because muscular harmony is the first thing to go astray once the spine starts feeling pain.

Hence, we follow a few fundamental exercises aimed at achieving three specific goals:

1. relaxing the over-protective hold of the long muscles running down either side of the spine
2. strengthening the abdominal corsetry so the tummy and back muscles make a strong, flexible torso to support the spine
3. re-educating the small muscles that control the individual spinal segments, so that bending is made secure.

These exercises are described in detail later in this section, along with a few mobilising exercises to help the BackBlock decompress the spine.

Back pain is often associated with a posture of the low back that is at variance with the norm. It may be too scooped out, or hollow, (called a lumbar lordosis) or it may lack any hollow at all so that it is completely flat. It may even curve the other way (the lumbar kyphosis). To redress these postures you may need to call on other exercises to bolster the work of the BackBlock.

Back pain associated with an over-hollow low back is usually caused by overloading the facet joints. In this position, they take too much weight (much more than the average of 16 per cent of load passing through the segment) and they grind under the strain. The pain usually worsens if you deliberately extend or arch backwards, in effect increasing the jamming.

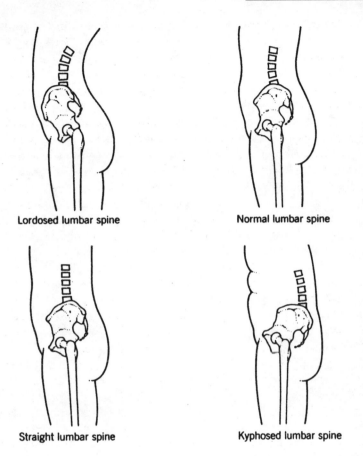

Lordosed lumbar spine

Normal lumbar spine

Straight lumbar spine

Kyphosed lumbar spine

Figure 6.2 Postures of the low back.

But often flexion or forward bending is just as painful because the incredibly strong facet capsules have become accustomed to the spine always being arched one way, and have adaptively shortened. The gentlest exercise for this problem is rocking the knees to the chest, on the floor, to open up the back of the spine. The best strengthening exercise is sit-ups.

Sit-ups should really be called curl-ups because that is exactly what they are. To prevent a shearing strain across the low lumbar segments you must 'curl up' rather than 'flip up' to the sitting position. *You must have your knees bent*, at first with the feet secured (under the bed or sofa), then feet unsecured as you get better at doing it.

The aim is to try to achieve controlled segmental movement where, like the cogs in a wheel, one vertebra after the other lifts off the floor. Always come right up to the fully curled position – chin on knees – and then down again in the same cat-curling, controlled fashion.

By the way, the real enthusiasts claim your tummy muscles will only work properly if you eliminate any contribution from the powerful hip flexor muscles. To do this, push your heels into the floor as hard as you can as you sit up. It is worth noting that sit-ups done by flipping up rather than curling may have some contribution from the back muscles, which ideally should be inactive. This may explain why back pain sometimes gets worse after doing stomach exercises incorrectly.

However, heels into the floor is too hard for me. And I fear the average sufferer will flail around on the floor stranded, like a beetle on its back, getting absolutely nowhere doing curl-ups this way. But by all means try if you can.

Sit-ups help by building up the strength of the stomach, the retaining wall at the front which straightens the sagging forward spine. This improves the 'resting posture' of the spine and reduces postural strain.

Whenever we bend forward – our most frequent, expansive and

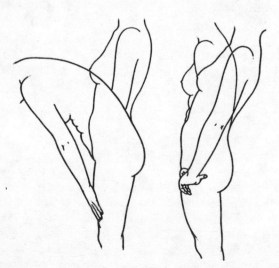

Figure 6.3.1 Pain associated with an increase in the lordotic curve is often relieved by curling forward.
Figure 6.3.2 Pain associated with a lack of normal lumbar curve (or a lumbar kyphosis) is often relieved by arching backwards.

precarious movement – a strong tummy helps the spine keep its column of segments secure as we go over. In the early stages of bending, the lower facet joints slightly disengage, thus leaving the segments appreciably more vulnerable to both forward shear and torsional strains. A strong tummy keeps everything in check.

However, it is the small, almost incidental movements before the tummy muscles start working that often cause you to rick your back. You can prevent this from happening by working extra hard on your muscle control – so, do those curl-ups. Remember, though, that it's important to do them correctly, otherwise you will damage your back. If you sit up with a jerk and without using the proper segmental curling action, the lack of holding power of the small muscles may allow the lumbar segments to shear forward, giving you a nasty new pain.

It is all too common to see sit-ups being done badly; it makes me wince to see the Rugby squad out there on the field, all doing their crunches and double leg-lifts. On the other hand, it makes me think that it won't be long before they all need treatment.

Quality, not quantity is important with sit-ups. You should aim for fine segmental control, so they must be done in a gentle, disciplined way. Eventually you should easily be able to do thirty sit-ups with your hands behind the head, knees crooked and feet unsecured.

Never attempt double leg-lifts, where you lie flat on your back on the floor and lift both legs. They are taboo! They create immense back strain because the effort involved causes the spine to arch perilously. There is really only one tummy exercise worth doing and that is the one described.

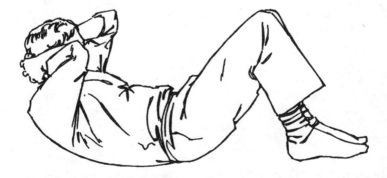

Figure 6.4 Sit-ups should always be done as curl-ups, although in the early stages you can do them with your arms stretched forward, instead of behind your head.

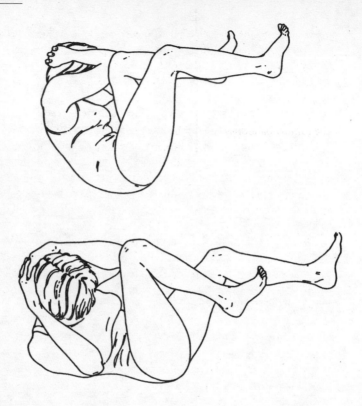

Figure 6.5 Pure oblique sit-ups.

The chief architects of perfect curl-ups are the *transversus abdominus* and internal and external oblique muscles. The obliques wrap around the abdominal wall, below the ribs and above the two ear-shaped pelvic bones. The fibres of the external oblique run in an inward and downward direction following the line that your fingers take when shoved inside a pocket. The internal oblique runs in the diagonally opposite direction, from the base of the rib cage at the front, out and down to the large hip bones. By acting in tandem in contrary directions, these two muscles make an 'X', thus creating an hour-glass waist. As with all muscle contraction, the fibres shorten in length, bending the torso across its middle to create the perfect sit-up.

This action significantly increases the intra-abdominal pressure, which in turn elongates and stiffens the links of the lumbar spine within the abdominal cavity. This partly explains the therapeutic value of this exercise and I can certainly vouch for its efficacy in my own clinics. Pure oblique action involves pelvic rotation as well as creasing across the abdomen. To do this you need to lie on your back on the floor, knees bent in the air. Difficult as it is, attempt to bring the right shoulder and elbow up to touch the left knee.

Sit-ups done badly are a disaster. The hip muscles do all the work, while the tummy balloons out and the compression effect on the spine is terrible. It is rather like creating bend in an unyielding flag-pole by increasing the tension on its stays. Eventually the pole bends, but at the expense of impacting it deeper into the ground. Hip flexors do the same thing to the spine. They compress the 'pole' and bring about angulation by pulling it forward at the hips. And for most spines, even uncomplaining ones, this is not a good thing to do. It drastically increases basal compression.

The difference between a good and a bad sit-up is critically important. Immense care must be taken to do them well. If you are having difficulties, help yourself up to the sitting position as best you can by pulling on your thighs (without jarring!), but once there, let go and curl back to the floor unaided. Emphasise a controlled return from the full curl, with your navel sucked in.

If pain prevents you from doing sit-ups, try doing hanging abdominals using a chin-up bar – it's an ideal alternative. Mind you, these have their difficulties too, especially for your arms and hands.

Stainless steel chin-up bars are available from most sports stores, and you can assemble them yourself on a door-jamb at home. Make sure the jamb is solid enough to take your weight and that you wedge in the bar very tightly so there is no danger of it giving way.

Grasp the bar firmly, preferably with gloved hands to prevent blisters. Let your legs hang free in mid-air. If the doorway is too low, you may need to bend your knees and tuck your feet up behind you. Using the principles of curl rather than flip, slowly but surely bring your thighs from vertical, right up to your chest. It is exceptionally hard work. You will never get your knees up under your chin but try to move in that general direction. At first, you will only manage two or three lifts and then your arms will give out. But hanging abdominals are valuable. They use the trunk-curling muscles without risking spinal compression and shear. There is even some pleasant separation of the lower joints as you hang there – all the benefits of abdominal exercise with a few others thrown in.

If frank degeneration of a disc follows on from thinning, it is because the nucleus has broken down and cannot disperse pressure. The nucleus

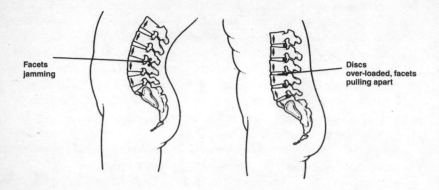

Figure 6.6.1 With an advanced lumbar hollow (a lordosis), excessive weight is taken through the facet joints as the back of the spine pinches together.
Figure 6.6.2 With insufficient lumbar hollow, too much body weight is taken through the vertebra-disc-vertebra strut of the spine (otherwise known as the neuro-central core).

becomes gluey and fibrous and, most important of all, flattens out on pressure instead of rebuffing weight. This subjects the interior disc wall to permanent assault from the runaway nucleus.

Small chinks start to open up in the inner layers of the disc wall which ultimately allow the nucleus to track outwards. Instead of behaving like a resilient spring, the disc behaves more like a perishing car tyre that barely keeps the weight of the vehicle off its rim. In the case of the back, the problem disc squashes with pressure and the flaccid walls distend, particularly when the spine bends forward.

With an acute flare-up of a disc, you will commonly find yourself fixed just a few degrees short of the 20-degree mark, unable to go any further forward because you will maximise peak bulging. But you may find it just as difficult to get back into an upright position because the bulge at the back of the disc cannot suck itself in as you roll back over it.

For this type of back there are two valuable exercises. They must both be done lying down so that the intra-discal pressure is at its lowest and the bulging least.

The first exercise is *passive extension*. This is done lying in the face-down position. At the outset, you may find it difficult getting into this position. You may be in a lot of pain and it may be necessary to place a pillow (or two) under your tummy to safeguard your bentness.

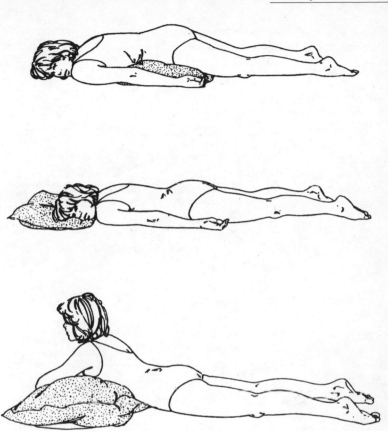

Figure 6.7.1 While you are still bent with pain, you will need to lie over pillows stacked under your tummy to get comfortable.

Figure 6.7.2 Slowly and progressively remove pillows until it is comfortable to lie flat.

Figure 6.7.3 Then you will stack pillows under the rib-cage to ease your spine gently into an arched position. This may take several hours.

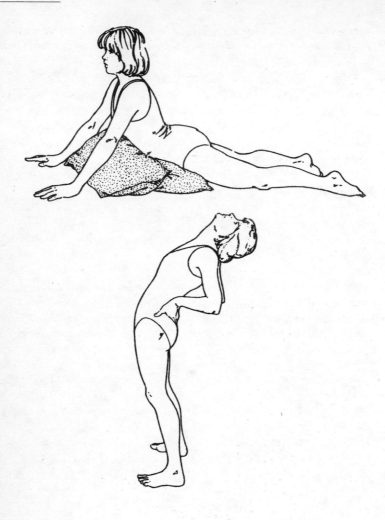

Figure 6.7.4 With progress, you will be able to arch the spine by pushing up onto straight arms. 'Hang' in this position for several seconds.

Figure 6.7.5 Eventually, in the standing position, you will be able to do a grand spinal extension, a much-needed release for the average spine. This should be avoided if back pain is associated with an increased lumbar lordosis.

But if you just lie there, you should eventually be able to do without pillows. It's easy to see why we call this exercise passive: you do nothing at all except lie there, letting gravity flatten you out straight.

By encouraging extension, we reduce the pressure on the disc by putting the facet joints in a better position to take weight. This also encourages the nucleus to squirt to the front of the disc, thus reducing the distortion effect on the back wall. As you find it easier to straighten out, elevate yourself onto your elbows and stay there for a minute or two, then lower yourself down again to a resting position. As this gets easier, push yourself up on both hands so the arms are straight and your spine drops down into an arch. Although this exercise may feel quite uncomfortable in the back, you should only be concerned if it worsens the pain in your leg. If it does, stop and just go back to lying peacefully on your tummy on the floor. If it is too painful to lie on your tummy, then just lie in any position you can, until you are in a less painful state. This may take days (see 'Should I Not Rest in Bed?' Chapter 4).

When you are in a much fitter state and can painlessly push yourself back into arched extension off the floor, then you should progress the exercise by doing the same in the standing position. Legs planted well apart with the fists thrust into the small of your back, lean over backwards. Do this several times a day.

This exercise is also useful if your back lacks a proper lumbar hollow. It helps to better distribute the weight of the upper body, which, by being

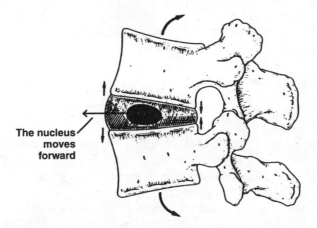

The nucleus moves forward

Figure 6.8.1 In extension, the nucleus migrates away from the back wall of the disc.

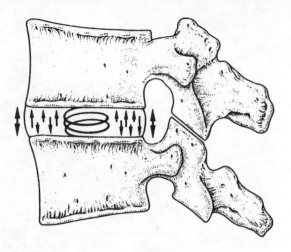

Figure 6.8.2 The combination of a healthy nucleus and the elastic lattice make-up of the disc wall means the whole disc acts like a coiled spring which resists compression.

carried too far in front of the centre of gravity, can cause a low back problem to develop.

As well as encouraging the nucleus of the disc to migrate away from a battered and bulging back wall, this exercise also stretches the spine back on itself and pulls out the very stout anterior longitudinal ligament, running down the front of the vertebral bodies.

When the spine has been immobilised for a long time through pain, the soft tissues that clothe it adaptively shorten. In addition to the circular disc wall clamping down, these contracted soft tissues exert a suffocating tethering effect on the spine and keep it permanently bunched down, disabling the spring effect of the discs.

Stretching the walls out again and freeing them from the restrictive soft-tissue binding, liberates the spring properties of the disc and this is where the *flexion* exercises come in.

Disc thinning, which is the precursor of most spinal problems, is reversed by all-round stretching of the disc wall. The wall itself is composed of twelve to fifteen concentric layers or thinner walls (called lamellae), the alternating layers of which have their fibres arranged diagonally at right angles to one another. This results in a tough, circular lattice around the rim of the disc which glues the segments together and also keeps the central nucleus contained under pressure. When the disc loses water and

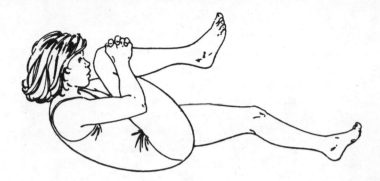

Figure 6.9.1 To open out the back of the spinal segments, gently pull one knee to the chest and bounce it there.

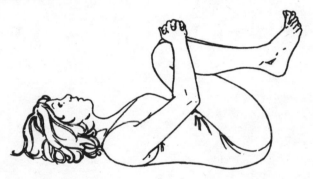

Figure 6.9.2 Repeat with both knees. Relax the neck.

compresses, the fibres of the tubular meshed lattice flatten out and gum down closer to each other. This makes the disc 'duller'; a much less efficient shock-absorber and it can be very difficult to reverse. The wall is much harder to pull up and the nucleus at the centre of the disc cannot imbibe fluid and puff itself up. Extension exercises (particularly using the BackBlock because the spine is unweighted), open out the front of the spine while flexion ones open out the back.

Getting the spine to bend properly when it has not bent for years is often a tricky business – but that doesn't mean you should shy away from it. The secret is to take great care and take your time. But you must do it.

Initially the flexion must be done lying down, so the pressure within the disc is at a minimum. Lie comfortably on your back on your bed. Gather up one leg behind the knee with both hands, ease it to your chest and gently bounce it there. As the pain abates, progress by bouncing the knee harder and then gather both knees to the chest and oscillate them together. Then you are ready to start bending the spine from vertical.

A safer, slower route to introducing the spine to full flexion from the standing position is to squat. This is a sort of half-way house and is marvellously releasing (although it does nothing to improve the muscular control involved in bending; touching your toes does that). Squatting is the spine's natural decompressor. Various indigenous peoples squat but we chair-sitters have almost lost the knack. We complain of strain in the knees and ankles, not to mention a strong pull in the lower back, but we often misread these signs. Although all stiff joints complain, they are inevitably enlivened and rejuvenated by squatting, especially the knees. Just try it.

Grab hold of the edge of the bath or some fixed support that can take your weight as you lean back. With your feet together and parallel and your heels flat on the floor, lower your bottom to the floor. Spread your knees wide with your outstretched arms between your legs. Now, bounce your bottom towards the floor, at the same time lowering your head forward between your knees. Do several bounces and then stand up, making sure to pull your tummy in hard as you rise from the floor. When you have repeated this several times, you will notice how the strain has lessened. In a week or two your knees will love it.

Incidentally, this exercise is excellent for disimpacting the spine when

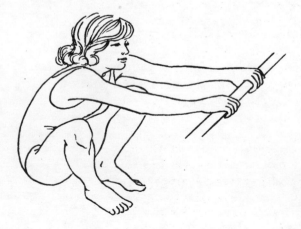

Figure 6.10 Squats.

you are out walking. If you start to feel your back becoming stiff and achy, use a low garden fence or gate and drop down for 10–15 seconds. It does wonders. Do your bounces and then continue with your walking.

The final progression involves bending forward from the standing position. It is normal to feel hesitant about doing this when the back hurts (especially if you feel a stab of pain in the early part of the bend), but it is imperative that you *do* learn to bend. You may need to start off initially by 'walking' your hands down your thighs (see 'Is Bending Bad for Me?' Chapter 8).

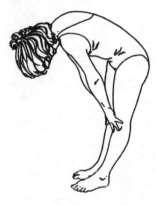

Figure 6.11.1 When you feel loath to bend, help yourself by climbing down your legs.

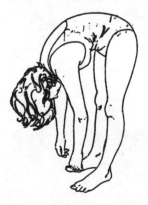

Figure 6.11.2 When you have arrived at the fully flopped position, relax and bounce carefully.

You must do the full bend, because that is where most benefit is. All recovering backs must do it. If need be, bend your knees slightly, so the back is not held up by tight hamstrings, and hang there like a gorilla. Carefully lower yourself into the full bend and stay there for several seconds doing tiny bounces. It becomes quite relaxing after a while.

Eventually, you can incorporate both flexion and extension into the same exercise. Lie face down on the floor, then push up on straight arms, hands on the floor below your shoulders, so your back hangs in a deep hollow. (In Yoga this position is known as The Cobra.) After a few moments, lift your bottom up and back and sit on your heels, fully curled forward, forehead on the floor if possible. (In Yoga, this posture is known as The Pose of the Child).

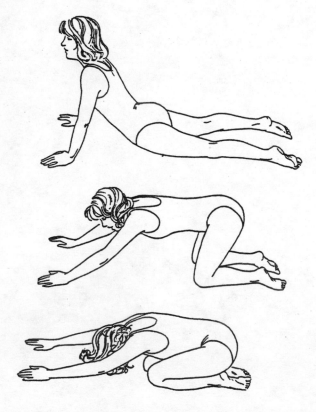

Figure 6.12 Cobra . . . through to . . . Pose of the Child.

In the starting position, you hang prone between your straight arms, pubic bone on the floor and taking care that your shoulders are not up around your ears. Hang there, breathing quietly as you relax. The spine should feel safe as the hips sink closer and closer towards the floor. After 15-20 seconds in this position, lift your hips away from the floor and back towards the feet, eventually sitting with your bottom on your heels. Now lower your chest to rest along the thighs, your face turned and your cheek on the floor. You can either put your arms to rest by your side, or you can leave them outstretched in front of you, ready for the return phase of the exercise. As you improve, you can do a rhythmic see-sawing action, passing from full hang to crouching back, each time feeling the back let go more.

However, you will always get a better separation of a stiff, impacted spine if you first subject it to a twisting stretch.

The best twist, done with a straight leg, is accomplished by taking up a position on the floor with lots of space around you. Lie on your back with your arms stretched out at shoulder level, palms down. Now, bring both knees up high onto your chest and then let them roll over to the left to rest, if possible, on the floor. As the knees go over, avoid letting your other arm and hand lift off the floor; this stretch usually gives a delicious pull across the front of the shoulder and chest wall. Then, finally, straighten the right leg at the knee and take hold of the foot or the ankle in your left hand.

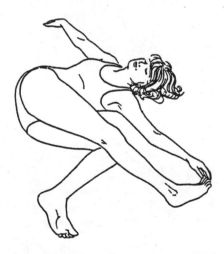

Figure 6.13 The floor twist.

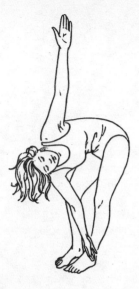

Figure 6.14 The standing twist.

By this stage, you will not only feel the pull in your upper rib cage and shoulder but also in the back of your right thigh and lower back. Hold the foot there and try to relax, breathing deeply as you feel the chest and leg let go. Since most lower back problems afflict one side more than the other, you will inevitably find the twist more difficult one way than the other. Ideally, you should repeat the exercise more frequently to the problem side.

To help the upper part of the spine (more at waist level and above) you can do a standing twist. This is done by standing with both feet flat on the floor, approximately 20 cm from the wall. Lean back against the wall so your bottom rests against it and then bend down, tightening your tummy as you go over. Let your right knee bend at will, at the same time taking the back of the right hand past the outside of the left ankle. At the same time, twist the torso and take your left hand back at the shoulder and high above your head, turning your head to look up at your thumb. As you stay in that position, keep the tummy well sucked in and, with each expiration, attempt to twist a little more. Always repeat the exercise, first one way then the other.

Another twisting stretch can be done while you sit in the office or in the car, although it is easier if the seat has arms. Start by pulling in your tummy and lifting your spine up out of the pelvis. Then, turn as far round to the right as you can go, while keeping your bottom on the seat. To give yourself

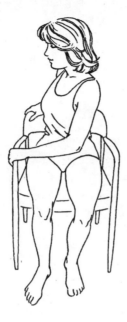

Figure 6.15 The chair twist.

more twist, lift yourself with your hands resting on the arms of the seat. When you have reached your perceived limit, pull your tummy muscles in a couple more notches and twist yourself further around. You will be amazed how much farther you can go. Always repeat to the other side. This exercise is useful because it can be done anytime during the day, whatever chair you are in. It greatly helps to puff up flattened discs.

The next aspect of this chapter deals with joints in the near vicinity of the low back which, by their abnormal function, may prevent the low back from returning to its former problem-free state. In this respect, the muscles and ligaments of the hips have the greatest role to play.

In the case of a lordotic lumbar spine, it is common for the hip flexors to be tight as well as the low back extensors. At the same time, the tummy will probably be weak, as will the muscles of the buttocks.

To stretch the hip flexors, lie on your back on the bed, letting the leg nearest the edge hang off so the hip falls back. Then, holding behind the knee, pull the other leg up to the chest and bounce it there gently. Repeat the same procedure with the other leg. As the hip flexors get more stretched, you could ask someone to exert pressure on the thigh of the straight leg to increase the force (see Figure 6.16).

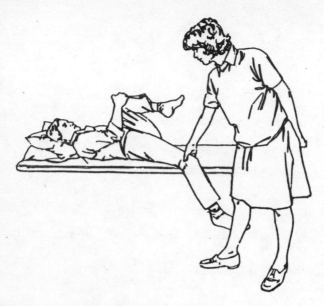

Figure 6.16 The hip-flexor stretch for the right leg.

The easiest way to stretch out the tight low-back muscles is to lie on your back and roll into a ball. Do this by holding both thighs behind the knees, linking the forearms if necessary. In this position, pull the thighs closer to the chest so you feel a stretching sensation in the low back. Don't be afraid to feel this pain – it is only beneficial (see Figure 6.17).

Statically pulling in your tummy and nipping your bottom in at the same time will swivel the pelvis under and take the hollow out of your low back. This is a subtle movement which you should try to do regularly throughout the day. At the same time, you should try to walk 'tall and light', so your spine hangs down from your skull in its optimal 'S' curve alignment.

If you try too hard to pull your tummy in, your shoulders will droop. Think about walking tall and moving freely. With the help of the newfound strength of the muscles that count, as well as the new freedom of muscles that formerly would not let go, you will find it easier to hold a more satisfactory stance (see Figure 6.18).

Various postural anomalies can be given a huge correctional boost by using a BackBlock. You can restore a proper lumbar hollow where a back habitually slumps in a reversed lordosis (lumbar kyphosis). Here, the BackBlock effectively pushes your bottom in as you lie over it on your back.

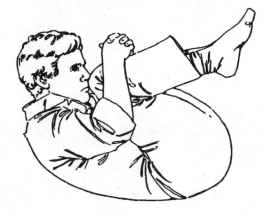

Figure 6.17 Rolling into a ball to stretch the low back.

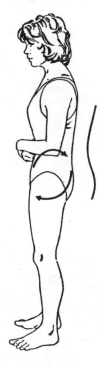

Figure 6.18 You can reduce an over-arched low back by nipping the buttocks under and rolling the pelvis back.

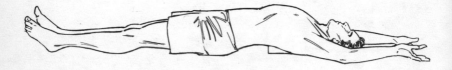

Figure 6.19.1
The BlackBlock under the upper back can cure a round-shouldered
posture and re-align the upper body over the spinal base

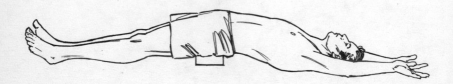

Figure 6.19.2
Apart from decompressing the spinal base, a BlackBlock
under the sacrum (at the back of the pelvis) can reduce
an over-arched low back and also re-align a too-
rounded low back

At the same time, it stretches the structures down the front of your spine (particularly the extraordinarily strong anterior longitudinal ligament) which, through shortening, have kept your body bowed forward. You can also lessen a lumbar hollow if that is too pronounced. Initially here, the BackBlock seems to accentuate the hollowing as the low back arches up more. But, as the hip flexors stretch (which goes with the pulling sensation across the front of your hips), there is an incremental backward glide of the lumbar segments which gradually lessens the hollow.

Using the BackBlock under the upper back (flat and lengthwise with the upper end level with the top of the shoulders) also helps to open out a hunched upper back. Moving the arms in wide semi-circles with the backs of the hands on the floor (from above your head down to your sides) also helps to stretch tight pectoral muscles which tether in the front of your chest and keep you hunched.

Having prised the spine into better alignment, strengthening *must* follow to keep the correction. To help reduce lumbar hollow, you must do sit-ups (see Figure 6.4), but to accentuate lumbar hollowing, when the low back is too flat (or humped), you need to increase the strength of the long back

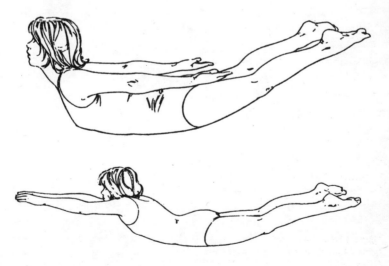

Figure 6.20 The back-arch can be done with the hands beside the body initially, then progressed to hands stretched above the head.

muscles to help hold the shoulders back. To do this, lie face down on the floor and lift the head and shoulders back in an arching action. This is quite easy to do and you should progress fairly quickly to incorporate lifting the arms, stretched out above the head. When that is achieved fairly comfortably, you should incorporate the legs as well. Work up to doing 10 backward arches (see Figure 6.20).

If you sit and stand in a permanent slumped position, it will make you very tired. This is because the spine cannot stay upright effortlessly and requires constant muscle action to keep the segments stacked aloft in a gently swaying pillar. The combination or re-alignment *and* strengthening rapidly makes life easier, and you will quickly feel less postural strain during your upright hours.

With their new-found strength, the long spinal muscles running up the back can reduce the tiring mechanical leverage of the heavy upper body being carried too far forward in front of the line of gravity. They pull the head and torso back into a less stressful position, aligned properly over the centre of gravity. Thereafter the back sits stacked happily upon itself, well supported from below by the spine arching gracefully down in its natural spinal curves. That tired aching disappears.

Another important mobilising exercise to optimise lordosis and un-gum the facets of a too-slumped lumbar spine is sustained stretching in the prone position. This is done lying, face down, on the floor with pillows stacked up under your ribcage; this gently brings the spine around into an unaccustomed hollow and forces the facets into a closer-packed position. Stay there for several minutes every day and when the going gets easier, progress to pushing up on extended arms so that the spine adopts a greater hollow. Eventually this should be done while standing by thrusting both hands into the buttocks and bending over backwards (see Figures 6.7.1–6.7.5). Effective as these techniques are, they are usually better followed by comprehensive use of the BackBlock, just in case the vertical over-arching has jammed the facets too much.

In a simpler form, it can be useful to lie prone in bed for a while before you go to sleep. The whole skeleton loves this welcome change from a day spent hunched over in studied concentration, and it helps redress the postural imbalance. But be careful not to stay there for too long – otherwise you might get cast rigid – and remember to wriggle your hips gently from left to right to loosen your back before changing position to get up.

Another exercise for releasing the fixed abnormal posture of a flat (or humped) low back is the hamstring stretch. When tight, these muscles,

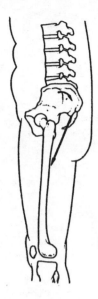

Figure 6.21 Short hamstrings will pull the pelvis around so that the spine humps.

which attach to the back of the pelvis, keep it rotated in a backward direction and roll the low spine into a hump (Figure 6.21).

The least stressful way to start this exercise is to lie on your back on the floor and bring one knee to your chest. From here, straighten the leg by pushing the heel towards the ceiling. You must lead with the heel; it's also important to stop the pelvis on the other side rolling back as the tension increases in the muscle.

When you have achieved a reasonable degree of stretch (which takes a week or so), doing a minute or so each day, then progress the exercise by doing it standing up. Find a low surface such as a foot stool, standing about forty-five centimetres off the floor. Support the heel of your action leg on the stool and, with the leg straight, bend your head down towards that knee. Do not allow the knee to flex and do not allow the pelvis to twist away from the action leg. Do these stretches once a day for two weeks and be sure to progress it by raising the level of the support as soon as the tightness eases (see Figures 6.22 and 6.23).

There is one instance where strengthening the spine itself is of value. This is where a segment in the spine has become loose or weak – the 'unstable segment'. This type of back is like a broken reed. It keeps folding

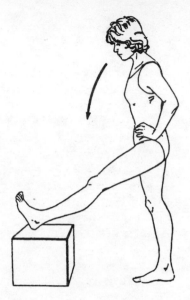

Figure 6.22 The first phase of a hamstring stretch of the left leg. Attempt to bring the nose towards the knee.

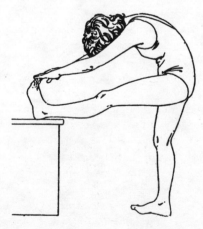

Figure 6.23 A progression of the same manoeuvre using a higher supporting surface.

up under pressure or when caught by an unguarded movement. In this case it is important to strengthen the weak link and bind it back together with good, strong muscles.

A significant feature of a spine harbouring a weak link can be seen by the way you get up from the bent-forward position. You find it impossible to go straight up, so you climb up your thighs with your hands in order to get upright. Equally typical is the feeling that your back will give way if you attempt to bend forward a few degrees, even over a washbasin.

As an intuitive protective reflex, you frequently try to reduce the shearing strain across the loose vertebra during recovery by tucking your bottom forward under the spine, so the lower joints are placed directly under the overhanging spine. Thus the centre of gravity is moved forward and straightening is made easier. This phenomenon is called 'reversed lumbar/pelvic rhythm' and it is useful as a treatment technique to familiarise spines with bending. This particularly applies to spines that haven't bent for years. And, as we shall see, if a back is to be completely healthy, it must bend, no matter how insecure it feels to start with.

When learning to bend, it is always preferable to do it in reverse first. This means lowering yourself down the legs, hands on thighs, to the fully flopped-forward position, and then rising, using the back alone without

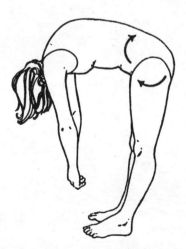

Figure 6.24.1 The action of 'unfurling' to vertical from the fully flopped position is initiated by sucking the tummy in, tucking the bottom under and rolling the pelvis back.

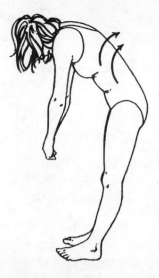

Figure 6.24.2 After the pelvis has fully rolled back, the spine uncurls to vertical.

help from the hands. When coming up, always pull in the tummy muscles and clench the buttocks to roll the pelvis back. This initiates the movement and, as a secondary action, the spine unfurls to vertical (Figures 6.24.1 and 6.24.2).

The 'long' back muscles, which are the obvious ones that feel like two ropy cords beside the spine, have no ability to hold the individual spinal segments in place. In fact, they do the opposite. They act rather like the stays of a flagpole. They keep us upright once we are up there. They keep the spine erect against gravity, but they exert no control over the individual vertebrae. This is the job of the small 'intrinsic' spinal muscles, which pass from vertebra to vertebra, keeping the segments snugly intact. They make sure each vertebra sits securely on the one below.

However, when the long back muscles are in spasm (which happens as a matter of course whenever the back is in a state of alarm), the over-action of these large, rope-like muscles reflexly inhibits the activity of the delicate, deeper muscles that control the finer movements. The bulky 'macro' muscles activate in one clumsy and sustained contraction, creating a bow-string effect on the spine. Conversely, the 'micro' muscles that master the intricate composite movements become inactive and the intrinsic stability of the spine is threatened.

If there is spasm – and you will always know because the back will feel unnaturally hard and stiff – the best way to get rid of it is by stretching it gently. The same applies with any muscle in cramp: you must gently elongate the muscle fibres that have locked up.

You can do this by lying on your back and bringing your knees to your chest, one leg at a time. When there, bounce them gently with small oscillatory movements (that is, not tugging them). You can keep your ankles crossed to make the legs less unwieldy.

The intrinsic muscles perform the invaluable role of stabilising the individual spinal segments. However, this is a subtle role and the degree of contraction of each muscle is not great. They are at their most active when unfurling the spinal segments from fully curled to an upright position. Once the spine is erect, it is relatively stable and the long back extensors then take over to hold it in place.

The way to strengthen these muscles, therefore, is to make them do just that movement. Lie face down off the edge of a secure table so that your torso above hip level is suspended in mid-air, head hanging down to the floor. Get someone to hold your legs and, from this position, slowly curl up from the base of the spine upwards, the head coming up last (Figures 6.25.1–6.25.3). Once again (as with the abdominal exercises), the emphasis is on individual segmental movement where one vertebra after the other comes up in a controlled way. The focus again should be on quality, not quantity. Aim to do 15 of these, but you may be prevented by the strain telling in the back of your thighs.

A universal 'best-seller' exercise, useful for just about every spinal problem, is the spinal rolling exercise. This is also done lying on your back. Gather both knees to your chest and hug them there. In this position, gently rock backwards and forwards along the length of your spine. The stiff link will be painful as you roll over it and you should concentrate on pivoting right there, worrying back and forth over it (see Figure 6.26).

The value of this exercise is that it passively mobilises each vertebra as your weight passes over it. In turn, each bone glides backwards. It should be done in a completely relaxed way so that you can keep the momentum going. It should have a mesmerising and comforting effect – most people do it with too much gusto.

If you are trying to localise the action to improve the functioning of L.4 or L.5, the two lowest vertebrae, you may need to straighten out your legs more to bring the centre of gravity further down the spine to where the problem is. The focus of the movement should be very small, otherwise you

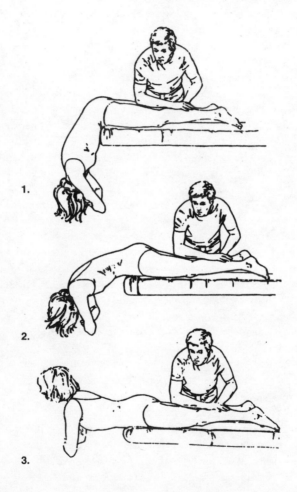

Figure 6.25.1 To improve the intrinsic strength of the spine, hang off the end of a high bench or table with the legs secured.

Figures 6.25.2, 6.25.3 By sucking in the stomach and rolling the pelvis back, unfurl from the fully dropped-down position up to the horizontal.

will spend too much time rolling over all the healthy vertebrae while achieving nothing at the trouble site.

As normality returns, you can start on more vigorous exercises such as toe-touching from a standing position. Ten bounces to the floor is about the right number.

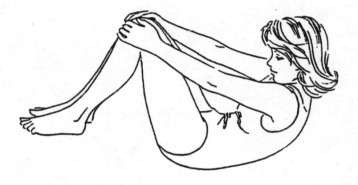

Figure 6.26 The best self-mobilisation technique is to roll the weight of the body back and forth over the problem link. In effect, you pivot on the problem link.

7 Sport and the Back

Today's world is sports mad. We are all led to believe that, with a bit more exercise, we would be superhuman. But truth is, some sports are downright bad for us.

Sport is good for heart and lung function. Blood races through the system, sweat rids the body of impurities, the lungs are exercised. But often the more physically aggressive sports are a hard grind for the joints.

The prime value of sport is *stretch*. The valuable sports do not decree monotonous, stereotyped movements as we see in tennis or golf, for example, but instead encourage spontaneous, uninhibited movement of unlimited variety.

Soccer is good because its reflex agility is spontaneous, compared to the studied precision, say, of ballet, and makes for an emancipated skeleton. Ballerinas often suffer bad backs for just this reason.

On the other hand, it is very bad for joints to have no exercise at all. They quickly tighten up and dry out. With total inactivity the bones de-mineralise and become brittle. You can see, therefore, what a bad idea it is to combine deskbound inactivity with bone-crunching sport. A stretching sport is fine, but not a bone-cruncher. In my view, parachuting and sky diving are among the worst because they combine such brutal impact after periods of inactivity. After all, there they sit, hunched up and cold, waiting for their aircraft to reach altitude; then they pile out, free-fall and land – crunch – through two legs which cannot hope to absorb such a shock. The spine telescopes into itself. No wonder so many devotees of these activities have back trouble.

Lots of sports are unnatural. Think about the awkward contortions of a hurdler, for example, bunching up and twisting over the gate, thumping down hard on the leading leg and then pulling the rest of the body over.

Table tennis, on the other hand, is excellent. It is quick and light. The playing area is small so there is a minimum of long run-ups with hefty thumping down on the floor. There are multifarious ways to swing and hit the ball, all of which involve stretching movements. The bat is small and light without unfavourable leverage. And it is extremely energetic. In no time at all you can work up a sweat.

Unfortunately, though, many sports over-use and abuse the joints. Too often they require strength rather than stretch, and strength invariably locked within repetitive patterns of movement.

Aggressive joint activity, back and forth within strict confines, wears out the joints and the harder you play a sport, the more trouble you store up for yourself.

The last item of bad news about sport is that, even if a sport does serve the requirements of stretch with only a modicum of repetition, it may still not have the qualities needed to cure your problem.

Usually sporting movement is not sufficiently careful to be therapeutic. It is unlikely to bring about the right movement at the right time, or the right degree of push in the right direction. It usually either bypasses the joint by allowing its neighbours to do the work, or it forces a stiff joint too far and hurts it. Sometimes, if a soft-tissue injury is in its final stages of recovery, it may be finally cured by going out for a long run or playing a gentle game of tennis. But, if it is not quite ready, this will provoke the problem anew and add to your troubles.

YOGA

Yoga is as clever as they come. It originated as long ago as 600 B.C. and exists today as a brilliant discipline of exceptional physical and mental subtlety. It is a collection of postures demanding stretch, balance and stamina. With its focus on breathing, it is gently calming and centring, which sets it apart from so many other forms of physical training.

The inherited flaw in the human skeleton is that all its joints tighten over time. The reason for this is twofold. Firstly, tissues lose fluid with age and, secondly, we use our joints without imagination. Not only do we repeat the same movements, over and over, but most of the useful actions take place within a meagre range of the joints' available freedom. This means that our skeletons all show the same pattern of mobility loss. We become like puppets with the same strings pulled too tight. Yoga helps in that it recognises the habitual way joints tighten and deliberately reverses each pattern. Take the shoulder for instance. As we get older, the first movement we lose is the arm going up above the head. However, that restriction will always co-exist with others you might not be aware of – in the shoulder's case, an outward swivelling action of the arm in the socket as it goes up.

What I am saying is that each 'functional' movement is made up of a composite of many 'accessory' movements that seem invisible. It is these movements, as integral components of the overall movement, which yoga brings back. A yoga arm-stretch, for instance, will always incorporate this hidden outward rotation movement of the arm in the socket A composite stretch incorporating accessory stretches will be much more effective than a simple stretch. Or, put another way, in a stretching regime, the quickest way to regain overall movement is a composite stretch rather than a simple one. In this way, yoga is much more sophisticated than the average aerobics or calisthenics workout. The yoga postures are beautifully designed to target many co-existing patterns of stiffness at the one time, working several joints at once. What is more, yoga highlights certain key problem spots (like the shoulders and hips) which, by their existence alone, are the cornerstones of more widespread trouble.

So, yoga targets incipient kinks in the skeleton before they become widespread and, by re-establishing background or accessory movement in all joints, it coaxes us back to health. Yoga also enhances high-performance co-ordination. It does this by facilitating 'fine joint play'.

Anyone employing so-called high-performance motor skills must have joints that can do what is needed of them. With the delicate work of the brain surgeon or the golfer sinking a hole-in-one, the co-ordinated effort of the muscles and joints is remarkable. To achieve absolute accuracy, the muscles must constantly make fine adjustments in the joints' angle of action. But they can only line the joints up optimally if each one is slack enough to accommodate this internal manoeuvring. The looser the joints, the more able they are to shuffle and adjust, and the more precise will be the ultimate performance. One reason for physical clumsiness is imperfect joint positioning. As we line up, poised in space to throw a dart or thread a needle, we can only do a good job if all our joints do a good job. Yoga keeps us in that optimal state of loosely active preparedness – and in getting us there, it winds the clock back and keeps our joints young.

So, yoga can not only make a super performer out of you by fine tuning the physical skills you already have, it can also stop lesser achievers from sliding backwards. It is preventative; it slows your deterioration and it is infinitely therapeutic. There is an enormous variety of postures from the very gentle to the immensely demanding. I advise supervision until you are well initiated and then you can do things on your own at home. (See my book *Body In Action*.)

JOGGING

Running and its milder version, jogging, are a great release but they do more for your mind than your body.

Those who jog feel an almost irresistible desire to get out and burn off energy, particularly after hours spent labouring over a desk. And indeed, running does have a calming effect. It puts you in a mind set where worries assume more normal proportions; solutions become clearer and take their rightful priority.

This can only help because, if left unchecked, stress has adverse physical effects. It is incredibly corrosive and undermines the body's health in many (sometimes sinister) ways. Stress particularly causes the skeleton to crack up. This is because the muscles never quite relax, even at rest, so that when you have something purposeful to do, they tire more easily. As a result, muscles often feel tense and sore and then additional strains happen with alarming ease.

The joints also suffer because they are cramped up under too-tight muscles. Their nutrition is reduced because the changes of pressure within the joint, corresponding to periods of strong physical work followed by lay-offs, are less marked. The blood stops flooding through the joint, as it does in the floppy, respite phases, and has to be squeezed through the permanently tensed tissues.

Strenuous physical exertion washes out stress. It seems that all reserves are called in and energy that was spent on anxiety is converted to physical output. Thereafter, it seems easier to relax, unwind and put life in perspective.

But although jogging is one of the best ways of clearing the head and releasing pent-up angst, it must be said that it is bad for the spine. It really bashes the joints around. Unlike walking – especially long, light, loping-stride walking where all the joints glide freely with minimal jarring – jogging greatly increases the stresses on the spine by piling the forces down through the body. As well as the spine, all the joints of the lower limbs suffer.

It helps if you run with a long-legged, fully stretched lope like the African marathon runners, because this increases the stretch of the hips and allows the low back to arch slightly to absorb impact maximally. The more elastic the hips, the better they, too, can absorb shock before it relays up to the spine.

It is important to note that when hips develop osteoarthritis (when the function of hip joints starts to deteriorate, simply as a consequence of our getting on in years), the first movement they lose is this backward or 'extension' movement. Running with long strides helps to keep the hips young by preserving this backward action.

A smooth, grassy surface is the least jarring for jogging; the smoother the better, with bumps and potholes presenting obvious dangers. The rubberised tracks of athletics grounds are also good. Their only drawback is that they permit absolutely no slide on impact. This can be very jarring, particularly for the hips. (Indoor netball/basketball courts exhibit the same problem.)

Whatever the surface, all jogging is greatly influenced by your footwear. Today there is an infinite variety of jogging shoes but the best are lightweight with thick, spongy soles, especially under the heel. Never jog in the old-fashioned plimsolls with their paper-thin rubber soles. The greater the shock-absorption qualities of the sole, the better the shoe.

However, having said all this, it would be neglectful not to dwell a little longer on the negative effects of running. Some of my most difficult therapeutic encounters have been to do with breaking the bad news about running.

Only now are we seeing joggers twenty or thirty years down the track, so to speak. Their skeletons are often appallingly gnarled, with problems developing at all the major weight-bearing joints. Their intellectual capacities may be in peak working order, but you should see their bodies! Joggers have to recognise that there *are* other sports which can bring the same benefits without the damage. It is often a partner who sees the warning signs. She relates how he gets out of bed and 'creeps around like an old man' until he has a shower and gets moving.

In the last few years I have become a lot tougher with runners. I no longer beat about the bush with them. If they accept my formula then I will continue seeing them, but the conditions are strict: a half hour of stretch, preferably yoga beforehand, the BackBlock and sixty curl-ups before running and BackBlock after, with toe touches at the traffic lights during the run.

TENNIS

Like lots of sports, tennis offers the skeleton a limited variety of movement. It consists of a series of hard smashes, all within the same few patterns of movement, using the same muscles over and over again. Like all repetitive sports, especially those which encourage fierce competition, tennis traps you in an exercise groove.

And while it may be exhilarating, and it is undeniably a pleasant, sociable game, it will not provide benefit, because its movements are so stereotyped.

At the risk of repeating myself, the general healthiness of joints is dependent on them having universal freedom to move fully in all directions. If they show a limited ability to go in any direction, it will not be long before pain sets in. Tennis has this major drawback.

Good sports encourage the skeleton to move every which way. The best are non-contact ball sports such as netball, basketball, soccer and table tennis. All of these provide a wide variety of movement and lots of stretch. Stretch is the all-important factor. Before any game, it is advisable to stretch the body, easing the joints out of their kinked constrictions. This balances the pull of muscles across the joints, and makes for greatly improved co-ordination during the game.

With tennis, its inconsistent energy output is a problem too, especially in doubles. The game often alternates between leisurely standing-about phases and explosive bursts while constantly waving a heavy racket in the air. There you are, standing in the middle of the court, thinking no ball can get past you when one comes lobbing over the net, just a little too short for comfort. You spring into action to make a lurch at it and – Bang! the back goes.

The racket is also a bit of a problem. Its length and weight create long leverage, which throws great strain on the spine, especially at full stretch; though this is more likely to affect the shoulder and neck part of the spine.

Tennis also involves a lot of running about on a hard court surface, which jolts the spine. The softer the surface (ideally grass), the better. Clay courts are hard but at least they allow players to slide a bit as the foot hits the ground, thus taking a lot of the shock out of landing.

However, any adverse effects of tennis can be partially minimised by using the BackBlock, ensuring that you have strong tummy muscles (sit-ups, again) and doing squats or toe-touches between sets. Bouncy, cushioning tennis shoes also reduce the jarring shock of landing heavily or lunging at a runaway ball.

AEROBICS

Aerobics is commonly taken up by the unfit in a frantic effort to get fit. In one quick session, people demand all sorts of things of their body which it may not have done for years, probably since childhood. And because the skeleton is not the fit, well-oiled machine it might be, it readily registers strain.

That said, aerobics is so much more useful than going to the gym, where the emphasis is on strength, strength and more strength. This difference is very important. Aerobics involves a good variety of stretch. In a good class, all the joints are targeted, one after the other, and the habitually tight ones, common to us all, are worked harder than the less troublesome ones.

The main risk with aerobics is 'too much too soon'. Many of the exercises are so physically demanding (both the stretches and the strengthening ones), that there is a high risk of strain, especially early on. Success depends on carefully stepping up the level of difficulty and endurance. If you get there without straining yourself, then you will be very fit indeed. It is a good way to keep fit once you are fit but it's not an ideal way of getting there.

The aim of aerobics, with all that frenetic exercising and running on the spot, is to increase the body's rate of oxygen uptake. As this increases, the level of fitness increases, and for this reason it is absolutely imperative to do your workout where there is lots of fresh air available. It is common and entirely counter-productive to swelter away with no open window or competent air-conditioning. Everybody staggers out feeling worse, rather than better, after one of these sessions.

SWIMMING

Unlike many people, I am not a great fan of swimming. I find it such a nuisance – going to a pool, undressing, swimming, showering, dressing, drying my hair, and so on – that the overall benefit is hardly worth the effort. A few specific exercises done at home are just as useful.

Swimming can even be bad for you if you have a backache that is made much worse by arching backwards – a problem usually associated with an increased lumbar lordosis. Swimming on your front has the undesirable effect of allowing your low back to sag, which immediately creates pain. People who can barely drag themselves out of the pool afterwards obviously have this problem.

In the face-down swimming position, the facet joints at the back of the spine close up and, if the joints are irritable, swimming freestyle or breast stroke can easily make matters worse. However, lumber disc problems often benefit from swimming because the neuro-central core (the central disc-vertebra pillar) is unweighted, thus reducing the intradiscal pressure.

On the other hand, free and languid body movement buoyed by the water brings undoubted benefits. The buoyancy makes it easy to move. However, strenuous kicking is not good.

Try following the typical hydrotherapy routine where you hang on to the rail running round the side of the pool at water-level height, with your back to the wall. In this position you can do free trunk movements and repeatedly bring your knees up to your chest. Do not do straight leg-kicks because this strains the spine. If you do swim, it is best to do so on your back as gently and rhythmically as possible, without straining.

GOLF

Unfortunately, golf is a one-sided activity. It repeatedly wrenches the spine one way as you take a swipe at the ball. Joints are healthy when they have a multi-directional freedom and golf does not encourage this. In fact, I cannot think of a sport offering less variety of action. Tennis, at least, has forehand and backhand strokes and the serve allows a nice throw into a full extension. Golf is completely monotonous.

All that standing about waiting for the other fellow to hit his ball isn't too helpful, either. The old tummy starts to sag. Indeed, as the spine settles into a deeper lumbar curve, it may become more and more difficult to bend over to get the ball; or, alternatively, your back may feel fine while you are playing but when you try to get into the car afterwards, you can hardly bend to do so.

As the spine becomes cast by the standing around, the frequent bends to pick up the ball are often done badly. So often we see a golfer bend like a geriatric granny, the legs planted wide apart, abdomen lowered down between the thighs and a stiff, arched spine tipped forward by bending at the hips. The resultant shearing strain across the lower lumbar joints is enormous and one often sees a protective hand fly unconsciously to the back to brace it for the inevitable stab of pain. Bending is so much more 'useful' (not to mention painless) if it is done as a proper curling action helped by a restraining hand to brace the tummy at the front.

Strong tummy muscles are a must for golfers. They prevent the forward sag of the spine while standing and they prevent the spinal segments from shearing as you bend to pick up the ball.

It is not uncommon to start feeling stiff on your way around the course. The best way to cope with this is by doing copious toe-touches all the way through the game. If it is too uncomfortable getting into a bend, squat on your haunches. This passively bends the spine around, stretching out your lower back and disimpacting the vertebrae.

The BackBlock plus loosening and strengthening exercises, done before and after a round of golf, will help keep you playing comfortably. You must also include twisting the trunk as thoroughly to the right as you would swing the club to the left or vice versa. Also, do put in some sessions of full and energetic back-arching to counter all that concentration and crouching over to putt. The best thing you can do is to throw yourself into extension and release those pent-up joints.

RUGBY AND SOCCER

Rugby is incredibly bad for the spine. Together with parachute jumping and sky diving, it is the worst activity for your back. Everything about rugby worries me for the skeleton's sake, although in truth, the neck probably suffers more than the back. But oh! how the joints get hurt. I can hardly bear to watch.

Imagine the impact on the skeletal joints of having one gigantic forward ploughing headlong into the midriff of another, both running towards each other as fast as their legs will carry them.

The other factor that contributes to rugby damage is the heaviness and muscular bulk of the average player. It is quite the opposite of the gazelle-like soccer player. Picture the way the soccer players leap through the air; no tackling, simply scoring points through light-footed co-ordination rather than by flattening some other poor chap.

Although it is true that larger men come off better after tackles, simply because they can bounce their assailants off, they often suffer because their bodies are too heavy for their joints. Their over-powerful muscles keep them bunched up and tight, not allowing full freedom. Yet more trouble in store.

8 Other Factors that Influence a Back Problem

It is often impossible to say what specific incidents trigger a back problem. We are all prone to trouble, whether we are secretaries or stevedores, musicians or removal men. Some of the factors that hurry on a latent back problem are discussed below.

AM I DEPRESSED BECAUSE OF MY BACKACHE OR IS MY DEPRESSION CAUSING MY BACKACHE?

Back pain is not easy to get rid of.

We all have only one back. If it is painful, you cannot use another while you rest it. It is on duty all the time, even during sleep, when it subconsciously turns us over or otherwise rearranges our sleeping position. And for every single, waking moment, the spine is at work.

For this reason, back problems can be long-term and relatively difficult to treat. There are more man-hours lost to the industrialised Western world through back pain than any other illness save the common cold. Treatment does not bring about instant cures. The longer the problem has been there, the longer it takes to fix. Living tissue can only rejuvenate at a certain rate and abnormal movement patterns take time to deprogramme. Good treatment (which includes disimpaction, mobilisation and muscle strengthening to re-educate trunk control and bending), combined with adequate rest and abolition of all aggravating factors, still takes time. It is a 'process', but it can be done.

If you are chronically depressed it is very hard to fish your back out of the mire. No treatment will work if you are beyond emotional reach; if you are so depressed you cannot even be raised to some expectation of recovery. You may have become locked in with your depression and your pain, each keeping the other going.

When we suffer from back pain, we are disabled; at times, it is impossible to think about anything else. It may be difficult to keep going, let alone 'achieve' or 'excel'. The very backbone of our ability is broken, and that is depressing. Pain is exhausting and, with no relief in sight, the future looks grim. Apart from the here-and-now anguish, the possibility that pain could go on forever is disturbing to say the least. The anxiety takes many forms, depression being the most common; and it hovers in the background like a dark cloud.

In practice, one sees many emotionally wrecked patients who are close to being destroyed by pain. At the time of their first consultation, one has the feeling they cannot be bothered to go through it all again. Replies to questions are glib and unemotional. They are convinced they cannot give any new leads by searching their minds for greater accuracy. Why should anything new succeed where everything else has failed?

The demeanour of people in permanent pain can be strange, with swinging mood changes. At times they can be frustrated and despondent, even insolent or hostile at the prospect of help. At other times they can be withdrawn or restrained, as if daring to let nothing out, lest the floodgates open and they dissolve, collapsed and sobbing, in a heap on the floor.

Usually, breaking free of the pain through treatment will restore you to your former self. The depression lifts as the pain fades and all atypical behaviour vanishes. You had simply been brought down by pain and, now it has gone, you are fine; optimistic, energetic and strong.

Sometimes, however, you and your therapist cannot banish the pain. It will be worrying for the therapist, who knows, by and large, from the way a back feels and behaves, just how much pain it will be responsible for. Of course, we do listen to the patient's testimony, and we do know that pain thresholds vary greatly. Even so, some backs just don't get better.

Perhaps you will continue to claim you have pain. You will continue to display the symptoms of depression, even though your therapist cannot find a valid physical reason to account for it. In these cases it must be recognised that a patient's unrelenting anxiety is perpetuating the expectation of pain – hence the pain continues. Sometimes the pain is entirely a figment of the imagination, although these cases are rare. Furthermore, even if it were so, one cannot say that the patient is not *'feeling'* pain. Pain is very subjective, impossible to measure objectively. One must believe a patient to be in pain if he, in his own mind, feels himself to be. Who is to say how much or little pain is imagined? And, if it is imagined, will it be any the less painful? It could be crippling.

Some patients grossly exaggerate their pain. They suffer a confusing degree of pain compared with relatively minor signs and symptoms. Back-ache is difficult to quantify. No passer-by can tell if you have it and sometimes we specialists are at a loss to know too. However, there is a small group of people in every community who actually derive benefit from having back pain. It is usually prompted by financial gain if there is litigation floating around in the background. And pain will never go away while lawyers are making more of it.

Making more of pain may also be prompted by a subconscious attempt to acquire attention or affection. He or she may feel that, except for their widely publicised back pain, they would be a faceless nonentity in the community. Alternatively, they may feel that the only way to rouse their partner from their indifferent torpor is to create a sense of pity or guilt.

Patients like these are extremely difficult to treat because the hidden agenda throws up impossible road blocks; they show no inclination to relinquish their pain. Some derive a perverse sort of pleasure from being unfixable; 'the nut that could not be cracked'; 'the back that dumbfounded medical science'. Their problem has become part of them and their lives have adapted to accommodate it. In these cases it is the families who need help, not the patient. Their numbers are few compared to the genuine cases, but it is these people who give the general mass of back sufferers a bad name.

DOES TENSION MAKE MY BACK WORSE?

Tension plays a very big role in spinal pain.

If there is a joint problem created by a recent injury, the pain comes from pressure within the soft tissues created by the trapped fluid. Such tissues have a characteristic puffy, swollen appearance.

If the problem is an older one, pain comes from perpetual stretching of the thickened or fibrotic tissues during normal functional activity. Either way, both problems mean the joint is tight to move. The two bones that make up the joint no longer hang together in a loose, shuffling harmony; the joint does not feel like a 'loose bag of bones'.

Tension can make matters worse by increasing the contraction of muscles surrounding a joint; in other words, tightening an already tight joint. Instead of the muscles being limp and relaxed when they are not in use, they remain 'tense', creating a further joint-jamming effect on the pre-existing tightness. This keeps the two joint surfaces pushed smack up against one another. Eventually the blood supply, and hence the nutrition through the joint, slows from a gush to a trickle. The joint becomes stiffer and more painful. Even fleeting bouts of tension jam up the skeleton, increasing the symptoms from problem joints. The husband who is accused of upsetting his wife and making her back pain worse has something to answer for!

Long-term stress is even more serious. This alone can make a problem joint out of a trouble-free one, simply by keeping it smothered under layers of permanently contracted muscles. The muscles ultimately lose their ability to relax, so there is incomplete recuperation after activity spurts and they tire more easily.

The mental spin-off of long-term stress is equally debilitating. Our judgement becomes impaired and our reactions inappropriate. We cease to see goals clearly and work towards them. Instead, we toil away in a middle-ground muddle, with no form to our day and no end in sight.

In this state, tension becomes corrosive; it gnaws away at health. Sleep becomes fitful and we are up, night after night, without the cleansing benefit of rest. We lose the resilience to throw off physical and emotional strains and, as our reserves go unreplenished, we run down. Disease creeps in as the body's defences are weakened by the long-term stress. The joints are the first to suffer but they are not the last.

SHOULD I LOSE WEIGHT?

Popular opinion maintains that you should lose weight if you want to lose your backache. Excess weight is significant but, in my view, it is not the be-all and end-all. The skeleton can bear weight without much complaint, especially the vertebral bodies. Bone itself is only very hard soft tissue: it is pliable and bends a lot during activity. The vertebrae sink and spring on top of their discs with every move we make.

In fact weight due to gravity, in combination with muscle activity, keeps normal bone healthy. Absence of gravitational pull on bone, as experienced by astronauts during long periods of weightlessness in space, has proved to be the most enduring problem for the scientists to crack. The decalcification of bones during space flight is exceedingly difficult to reverse; they cannot get calcium back into the bones.

The everyday significance of this means that normal gravitational stress on bone – which includes the natural heaviness of the body plus all sorts of running, jumping and standing-still activities – keeps the bones compliant and robust.

Conversely, absence of body movement or a gross reduction of body weight causes demineralisation of the bones. This makes them brittle and inelastic and unfortunately, if bone loses its spring, the joints jar more. A happy medium between heaviness and activity is the ideal; also, the joints will be slower to wear out.

While on the subject of calcium and the fact that movement makes bones stronger, it will come as no surprise that this relates to the healing rate of fractures. We have found that gently moving the two opposing bone fragments at a fracture site actually increases the rate of deposition of calcium within the soft plastic callus, the precursor of real bone. This means that the rate of fracture repair is faster and this is especially significant in cases of delayed union of a broken bone. It would seem the age-old tenet of total, immediate and lengthy splintage of broken bones in plaster of Paris may, in some cases, be redundant.

Back to weight again: if you are overweight, there are probably other factors involved which do cause harm. You are probably unfit. The muscle groups that control the spine (and the trunk) will be out of balance: some may be short, others long and most weak. The important groups, most particularly the tummy muscles, will have reduced strength and reduced endurance. Your skeleton will not be held trim and erect so you cannot effortlessly hold your belly in and your head high. Your thighs will be weak so you will have to haul yourself out of deep chairs or up flights of stairs.

In brief, you will move badly and in a sloppy fashion which is jarring for the joints. There will be 'postural strain' as you stand because everything starts to sag. As a consequence of inefficient movement, you will tire more easily. In fact, you will have such a job heaving yourself about that you tend to sit more – heavy, burdensome sitting in lazy postures which are bad for the back! The excess body load weighs down the skeleton and tends to accentuate bad postures. It is the poor posture that strains the joints, not the pure weight load.

After all, there are many fat but fit people. Look at those gargantuan Japanese sumo wrestlers for instance. They will have no greater propensity to backache than you or I, because these other factors of unfitness or pure laziness do not exist. It is therefore quite possible to go on being happily overweight if that is what you want, as long as the general body performance is raised to carry that load.

To recap, you may be able to minimise your backache by losing weight. It undoubtedly helps the situation but it won't rectify everything. To do that, you must clear up the mechanical problem responsible for the pain and then tone up the muscle support system holding the spine in trim. Thereafter you can stay as fat as you like – provided you don't die of a heart attack.

If you are overweight but manage to get a bit fitter, the improvement in strength and in heart/lung function will make it easier to do everyday things. The weight will then start dropping off, just because you are moving about and doing more. Unwittingly you will make yourself slimmer without even trying. This accounts for the common observation amongst dieters that, in the early stages of dieting, nothing seems to happen. Then weight loss suddenly gathers momentum without any appreciable change in the dieting format.

Dieting need not be so drastic if you combine it with more activity to burn off the weight. So many hapless dieters starve themselves to such an extent that they have little energy left to do anything. They drag themselves about all day, flopping from chair to chair, quietly getting fatter and fatter through lack of revs. It is a most unfortunate stalemate and a common state of affairs.

Dieters need to recognise one important fact: a reduced intake of food lowers the metabolic rate. This is an in-built precautionary measure to stave off disaster but it means that the less we eat, the less oxygen we consume and the less able we are to be active. Our activity palls because our 'fire within' fades and this leads to an increase in fat reserves. Beware of stringent dieting!

WHAT SHOES SHOULD I WEAR?

There are two important things about shoes: the height of the heel, and what the heel is made of.

The higher the heel, the more it tips the body forward in front of the line of gravity. As the pelvis is thrust forward, the low back must over-arch backwards to bring the weight of the upper body behind the line of gravity again. A higher heel can make all the spinal curves exaggerated. Pain is then never far away. There was a fashion for 'Earth shoes' designed with the heel lower than the forefoot. These employ the opposite principle to encourage better posture and a healthier spine. They are quite a good idea.

However, just as important as the heel height is its shock-absorption qualities to minimise impact when the foot strikes the ground. The softer and more rubbery the heel, the better. Crêpe rubber is best; wood is worst; and wood with metal caps under the heel is fiendish.

City gents do not like crêpe rubber soles too much. They don't go well with the pin-striped look. 'Sorbothane' sole-inserts are a good alternative. However, they do not go well in women's shoes, especially the higher ones, since the insert tends to creep down to the front of the shoe and gather under the toes. An insert may also make the foot ride too high in the shoe. (I insist patients with nasty back problems wear shoes with crêpe rubber heels during treatment, and thereafter if possible.)

SHOULD I WEAR A SURGICAL CORSET?

Except in rare circumstances, which I will describe in a moment, these contraptions are positively the worst thing you can do for your back.

If there is one message I have tried to convey here, it is that movement is therapeutic. Although it may hurt to move, there are good hurts and bad hurts. Most are good – and move we must. Movement begets movement. The more we move a joint, even a painful one, the better it moves. Pain is usually the result of poor mobility from malfunctioning joints.

I believe corsets came into vogue in a climate of desperation because we – all types of back treaters – could think of nothing better to do.

To encase the low back in a corset is a very short-sighted solution. It simply makes the spine stiffer, more brittle and more vulnerable; ready to be jarred more and more by trivial bumps and bangs. Spinal tolerance to shock is therefore steadily reduced.

The short-term gains of a corset are:

- A tightly worn corset can 'unload' the neuro-central core and thus reduce the intral-discal pressure on a problem segment.
- With acute inflammation, there can be initial pain reduction because the joint is kept quiet.
- A sagging belly is pulled in closer to the line of gravity, which reduces the forward drag on low lumbar facets.
- With severe spasm of the back muscles, a spinal support allows them to relax.

The long-term disadvantages of a corset are:

- Increasing brittleness of the spine.
- Weakening of the tummy muscles because they have so little to do.

The patient who arrives for treatment for the first time wearing an age-old corset is usually a tricky one to manage. For months, even years, he has been following advice never to leave his bed without it. He feels naked, vulnerable and frightened without it, sensing that his spine is too weak to go it alone. The sad truth is that he probably *will* do something to hurt his back because it has become so weak. He must be weaned from his corset, starting with an hour a day. Only then will he start getting better.

The spine has to be mobilised at any of its sticking levels and then it must be strengthened so it can bend. This is only possible by improving the

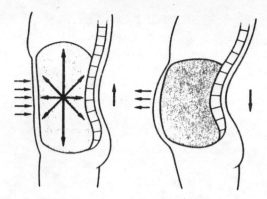

Figure 8.1 The bracing effect of a corset increases the intra-abdominal pressure, which 'lifts the spine up through the neuro-central core.

strength of the tummy and deep spinal muscles (intrinsics).

In circumstances where corsets do have a role to play, the benefits come from their tightness, not their rigidity; just like the kidney belts of weightlifters. These pull in the waist and greatly increase the pressure inside the belly. This 'unloads' the spine and reduces the risk of straining the back during heavy lifting.

Surgical corsets must do the same thing. The waist-belt must be hitched in very tight and the steel stays for inserting down the back of the corset should be thrown away.

IS BENDING BAD FOR ME?

No. Bending over in a deep, full sweep and up again is unquestionably the greatest treat you can give your spine. Bending keeps your back young.

The old directive of 'back straight, knees bent', faithfully carried out by hordes of patients, young and old, is the single most misguided, erroneous principle ever to be propagated. It simply perpetuates a stiff, brittle spine, *and that you do not want*. Besides, there will always come a time when you have no option but to bend – usually an emergency reflex action such as catching a falling cup. If your spine is not well accustomed to bending confidently, even a trivial incident such as this can cause havoc. It demands something that a brittle spine is not equipped to offer.

Of course, if you are to bend and lift something heavy like a suitcase, then it is better to lift like a weightlifter, with the back straight and bending the knees (see 'How Should I Lift?' later in this chapter). But for the average bend – to get the detergent from under the sink or to pick up a hand-kerchief from the floor – *you absolutely must use your spine*.

Bending gives the discs a drink. The nucleus inside the intervertebral disc consists of a colloidal jelly which attracts fluid. It is constantly trying to drag fluid (containing nutrients) into its midst to gain nourishment and this is greatly enhanced by full, expansive movement of the spine. With sitting down, standing up, stretching, twisting and bending, a squash-release-suck effect creates a two-way tidal flow of fluids in and out of the rich reserves of blood in the vertebral bodies above and below.

A variety of different bending directions is desirable because this avoids weakening the back wall of the disc, which could go on to form a focal bulge (a 'slipped' disc). On the whole, bending has suffered from a blighted reputation. Earlier schools of thought clung rigidly to the view that it was 'unnatural' and could pop a disc out. The fact that we have so long propagated this view is to our professional shame.

Patients confined to bed in hospital for non-back-related reasons lose disc-height, and x-rays taken before and after the confinement reveal this. Their discs, deprived of generous movement, effectively shrink from malnutrition.

Full and generous bending, because it is the grandest movement the spine has, keeps the ligaments and all the soft tissues supple and stretchable; it keeps the facet joints at the back of the vertebrae well oiled; it keeps the spinal cord free and slippery in the spinal canal and it keeps the spinal nerves elastic like strands of cooked spaghetti, free to pull out of the spine as the tension on the sciatic nerves increases.

Bending is a little more tricky if you are right in the middle of a flare-up of the back, particularly if you have been in trouble for some time and the deep muscles that control the individual segments have weakened (which they do automatically). Although it is imperative that you do bend, you must brace the tummy extra hard to prevent any slipping forward (called shear) of the vertebrae. The initial twenty degrees of tip should be done with care. The stomach muscles must be sucked in like a greyhound, even with a gently restraining hand, as you pass through the 'weighted-bending' phase.

Once the movement passes into the 'hanging' phase, where the segments are kept stable by the tension of the 'posterior ligamentous system' (the festoonery of ligaments down the back of the spine), the real benefit of the bend begins. The back of each interspace is opened out. This sucks fluid into the discs and also disimpacts the facet joints.

If you don't feel secure enough to bend, and you are worried the back will spasm, lower yourself down by climbing down your thighs, taking weight through your arms (see Figure 6.11.1, Chapter 6). When you are down there, hang. It matters not whether your knees are straight or slightly bent – as long as you really pull the spinal segments apart. As you hang there, make small, oscillating bounces. Return to vertical by sucking in the tummy, tightening the buttocks and rotating the pelvis under, then wind up to vertical from the base of the spine upwards.

If the back feels weak and threatens to give way, you can prepare yourself by bending it in a completely unweighted position, lying on your back on the floor and bringing your knees to the chest. But strengthening the 'intrinsic' back muscles (see Figures 6.25.1, 6.25.2, and 6.25.3, Chapter 6) is the all-important way of getting a back to bend. It provides the spine with much needed, almost instant strength, so that it loses that unnerving feeling of folding up and giving way whenever it leaves the vertical.

Bending over and staying bent, as in gardening, is another story. This is a strain. It is an impossible leverage for the muscles to cope with for any length of time and they soon tire and start aching with fatigue. This also stretches the soft structures of the spine too much, over too long a period of time. The more you return to upright, the less strain there will be. To garden, you should squat or kneel, ensuring the tummy is braced so the spine does not sag forward.

HOW SHOULD I LIFT?

Lifting in the workplace has done a lot to focus the collective mind on back problems, not least because of the cost to industry. Over the past decade or two, there has been much debate: what is a safe weight to lift, should we round the back to lift or keep it straight? In short, what advice can we give our workers to keep them in work and out of the law courts?

It's really quite amazing how a back can lift, bearing in mind what this means: bending a slender, multi-segmented column over double and then correcting to vertical, while at the same time carrying a load. Like a half-shut pen knife opening out straight again. Sensational.

The action is best understood by watching the techniques of professional weightlifters, because they demonstrate in a pure form what heavy lifting is all about.

The key factor in successful heavy lifting involves powerful intra-abdominal pressure, slightly humping the low back. As a weightlifter bends over to contemplate the weight, he signals the start of the lift by a deep, stout inhalation. This fills the lungs with air and causes the diaphragm to descend into the abdominal cavity. As the abdominal cavity reduces in volume, it increases pressure. This helps shore up the spine within and thrusts it upright.

This pocket of pressure under the diaphragm is exactly like a hydraulic sack, it buoys the spine aloft and unbends us from a curled position to an upright one. It is rather like a child's tubular paper whistle which un-bends as it is blown full of air.

The importance of intra-abdominal tone in a non-lifting state is well illustrated by the demise of poliomyelitis victims with paralysis of their trunk muscles. Because they lack tone, the torso gradually crumples down around itself. The muscles (the tummy muscles in a simultaneous co-contraction with the back muscles) are unable to build up enough abdominal pressure to push the spine aloft and the spine topples over. The result is an increasingly marked slumped spinal deformity.

Back to the art of lifting. When we are bent over to take the weight from the floor, the spine is relatively safe. It is locked by virtue of being at full, rounded stretch, with the posterior ligamentous system fully taut. All is set to take the first heave. The trickiest part comes when the weight is airborne and the ligamentous system develops slack. As the spine comes off full stretch, the vertebral segments can shift and shuffle under the burden of the load.

At this point, the successful lifter unconsciously prevents the spine from damaging itself by imperceptibly rolling his pelvis back, so the low back humps. In the process the stomach forcibly contracts and the low back feels like a strong, tense cylinder.

A poorly executed lift often fails at this stage, frequently resulting in a ricked back. As the load comes off the ligaments and is transferred to the back muscles, the spine flicks from a full stoop through to a full arch and it is at this point that the segments can squelch forward. This can be prevented by powerful, ballooning pressure from the abdomen below. With the spine now off the stretch, intra-abdominal pressure elongates it from within and stops it wobbling. This momentary phase 'rolls' the torso over a sprung spine, enabling the strongly contracting back muscles to take over safely.

Incidentally, recent understanding has paved the way in unlocking one of the chief mysteries of the lifting back and I need to explain this here. Mathematical calculations of torques and loads on muscles appeared to disprove the ability of a fine, streamlined human back to lift. Judging by the known muscle-contributors, it seemed that the power to straighten under load simply wasn't there! Then, the involvement of another two muscle groups was revealed. The *transversus abdominus* and the internal oblique muscles were observed to actually help straighten the spine and thus perform the opposite action previously attributed to them. As a result, some of the missing straightening power, over and above that provided by the long back muscles, was now recognised as coming from the unlikely source of the stomach or side-trunk muscles.

Their contribution is twofold. Firstly, they tighten transversely around the girth, thus pressurising the intra-abdominal cavity, which we know to be valuable. But more importantly, by their attachment to a lattice-like sheet of tissue (the thoraco-lumbar fascia), which in turn attaches to the backward projections of the spinal vertebrae, they assist directly in straightening the spine. As we will see in the section ('What is Wrong with Pushing'), by tugging laterally at the edges of this broad sheet of tissue, these two muscles cause the lattice to shrink in height as it is stretched out sideways. This has the effect of approximating, or bringing together, the individual vertebrae of the spine in just the same way as when we straighten. Far from tipping the spine forward and causing its small knobs to move apart as it elongates, the action of the muscles and the fascia draws the backs of the vertebrae together and straightens the back. Amazing!

The very same action of the human lattice regulates the free fall of the torso as we tip forward in bending. This again illustrates why nipping the stomach in with bending is so critical; it tenses the thoraco-lumbar lattice which retards the rate of the vertebrae pulling apart as they move forward.

It explains why serious weightlifters pay such close attention to stomach strength in their work-outs. They recognise that, without a stomach as hard as steel, they will not be able to lift effectively.

To revert to lifting in the workplace: with repeated heavy lifting, the intervertebral discs suffer the brunt of destructive forces. As we have seen in the section on disc degeneration and prolapsing (see Figures 3.3 and 3.4, Chapter 3), discs tend to suffer wear and tear at their left and right back corners. If we picture a disc as a clock face, most wear and tear corresponds to 5:00 and 7:00, where the disc rim is the most pinched by rotatory movements.

This is important because virtually every movement we make involves rotation. Movements of the human body are never pure. Even passing the salt involves a certain degree of twist. It gives us our own peculiarly 'living' way of doing things, as distinct from the mechanical up-down, left-right actions of a robot, for instance. It allows us to address objects face-on rather than at less manageable angles. This is particularly relevant to lifting. We

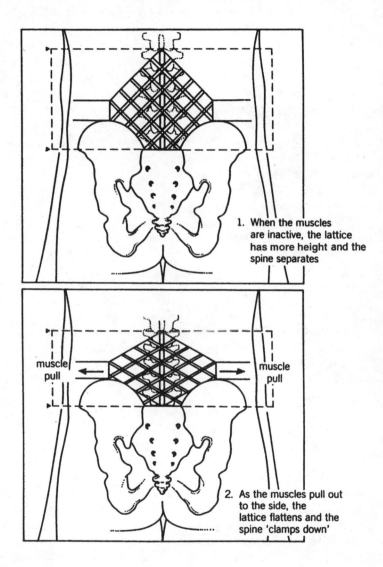

1. When the muscles are inactive, the lattice has more height and the spine separates

muscle pull

muscle pull

2. As the muscles pull out to the side, the lattice flattens and the spine 'clamps down'

Figure 8.2 The action of transversus abdominus and internal oblique muscles on the latticed thoraco-lumbar fascias.

have to bend to the side as we go down and come up, to get out of the way of our knees.

When we go to bend forward, there is a pay-out of the muscles on either side of the spine which act like large elastic cables, gradually letting go and allowing the spine to tip forward. Once we have grasped the weight we intend to lift, these same cables contract and help pull the spine back up to the straight position. This exerts compression on the spine, particularly on the discs, which tend to bulge out at the back. The back wall is even further subjected to assault if the central nucleus is partially degraded and has lost cohesion. This nucleus will squirt backwards against the inside of the rim, in effect, buffeting the back wall of the disc from within. If we combine the compression and the torsional strains of lifting, you can see that the forces of destruction on the discs are great.

That is why lifting in the workplace needs to be carefully controlled. As far as injuries are concerned – and contrary to conventional thinking – you are better off lifting with a rounded back, and then straightening the legs and back *at exactly the same time*. The critical factor is tummy strength. Another factor involves the closeness of the weight to the body; the further out from the body, the greater the strain.

In the workplace, lifting movements should be as varied as possible, bending down to the left a few times and then to the right. Try to intersperse the lifting routine – again as much as the working environment can accommodate – with some form of 'pause activity' such as spinal extension (see Figures 6.7.5, Chapter 6). If the job involves repetitive lifting in one way, then your pause activity should concentrate on twisting the other way. This is important, as it will maintain mobility of both sides of the skeleton, thereby reducing the likelihood of overuse and strain down one side. Pure side-flexion pause activity is often as helpful as rotation and spinal extension. This consists of standing, legs apart, and bending over sideways, running your fingertips down the outside of your thigh to below your knee. You should also try to avoid lifting directly from the floor. The height of the surface from which you lift is important. Generally speaking, the higher off the floor, the better, the optimum height being around elbow level. Any higher will mean that it is harder to get at and that the weight has to drop into your arms, posing the risk of jarring the back. If the object is heavy, you can brace your hip against the support structure and take it cleanly in your arms without undue strain on your back. The height where you off-load is equally important. Keep your stomach braced at all times and your eyes on where you are putting the load. If your lifting is heavy, repetitive and long-term, wear a kidney belt – or quit!

More people can carry medium weights, such as babies, than think they can. In fact, within reason, too many people with a back problem don't use it enough. A back will never be normal if you don't make it do normal things. A bit of lifting is very beneficial, especially if it is done in an unhurried and controlled way with the tummy braced. It strengthens the spine and helps break that stalemate of stiffness/weakness which is the greatest cause of ongoing trouble.

It may be useful to get into a stride or lunge position when lifting a medium weight. This means that you swoop down on to the weight and scoop it up, making the lift a full and dynamic movement, rather than a harried stab from above. A deep, lunging movement also means that the big joints such as the hips and knees, which are designed for load, are involved in the movement instead of just one willowy spine, working like a derrick from above. Keep the tummy braced and use the thighs!

It is quite possible that your back may be stiff and sore after some early lifting, but that is no bad thing. Don't be thrown by this and rush straight back to bed. The average back sufferer is too easily frightened by the worry of another 'attack'. This anxiety and the consequent tension can hasten one on, which otherwise might never have come. If the back is a bit sore after lifting (and it might well be), do some gentle rolling, some toe-touches and then some sit-ups (see Figure 6.4, Chapter 6). Then do some more lifting tomorrow.

Lifting an awkward weight, like lifting a heavy weight, also has its risks. For that reason there are a few fundamentals that you must follow. Ideally, get some one to help. Then, get right up close to the weight. Make sure that you get a good grip on the weight, and that your helper is going to lift at exactly the same time as you (lots of back injuries occur when the other fellow drops his end). Lift by straightening the knees and *at the same time* pulling in the tummy hard. Featherweights and light weights should be picked up from the floor with one full sweeping flowing action of the spine down to the floor and up again (see 'Is Bending Bad for Me?' earlier in this chapter) like a ballerina.

I know this flies in the face of just about everything you have heard about backs but just try it! Stiff, upright rigidity is dangerous. It's gotta go!

WHAT IS WRONG WITH PUSHING?

Pushing is a problem. There is no other activity more likely to cause even a normal back to break down. It can be something as absurdly simple as pushing a shopping trolley or mowing the lawn! The muscle that works rigorously during pushing is *transversus abdominus*. The fibres of this muscle wrap transversely around the sides of the lower trunk, between the bottom of the ribs and the top of the two hip bones. The action of the transversus is such that, as it contracts, it tightens around the waist like an elastic cummerbund. At the back of the torso, the muscle attaches itself to a broad, flat expanse of soft tissue consisting of diagonally placed fibres resembling a lattice (the thoraco-lumbar fascia). As its outer end is pulled taut by the contracting muscle, the lattice expands laterally but shortens vertically. Since the other end of the lattice attaches to the lumbar vertebra, it means that whenever the transversus abdominus contracts, the lumbar vertebrae are telescoped together. This is a superb piece of muscular enterprise. It means that whenever such a contraction takes place during bending or pushing, the spine 'clamps itself down' and resists forwards and backwards shear of its segments. The lattice steadies or tempers these otherwise risky movements by its compressing action. Sure enough, if you push hard against an object, you will telescope your spine and feel the side of your waist harden with the effort (and in a similar way, if you are in the garden raking leaves or grass, you will feel the abdominal wall tensing). The only hitch is that excessive effort in pushing may create too much telescoping and bring to light underlying spinal trouble. Pushing is often the last straw.

Unfortunately, the shape of the facet locking mechanism also works against the interests of the spine during pushing because it encourages spinal compression. These bony catches act in a way that locks them against each other when bending forward and this prevents each vertebra slipping off the one below. As we bend forward and until the lock engages, the upper vertebra slides up and forward on the lower vertebra. But when we do the opposite movement – which is what happens in pushing – the upper vertebra slides back and down the one below, bringing the two vertebrae closer together. Thus backward shear tends to jam the spine down upon itself.

And whatever is wrong with the spine – whether primarily in the front compartment at the disc-vertebra complex or the facets at the back – it will be aggravated by this extra compression. The discs will be further flattened and the facets will over-ride.

Incidentally, the reverse movement of backward shear – that of one vertebra being pushed forward on the one below – may account for the uniformly pleasing results of central mobilising pressures as a treatment technique (gliding the vertebra forward from behind), whatever other

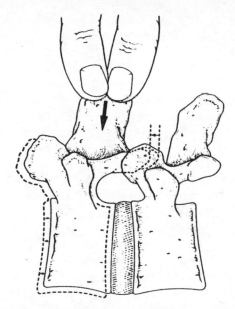

Figure 8.3 The simple 'sliding-up' effect of pushing on a lumbar vertebra in a postero-anterior direction. Two adjacent vertebrae are disimpacted.

movements the spinal segment lacks.

This manoeuvre, in effect, slides one vertebra forward on the one below, thus disimpacting the two bones as the upper one runs up the slope of the bony catch below. These 'central pressures', as we physios call them, are the single most effective therapy for painful backs.

The results from a few quick pushes and pokes to a problem vertebra are astonishingly good. And would the good Lord have made it any other way? Cavemen didn't have access to injections and image intensifiers, MRI machines and the rest of the shining armoury of chromium gadgetry. If a chap had a spot of backache, he probably got his mate to give his back a rub or maybe he even got him to put his heel into the painful spot, and that was that. Modern science has made us all too careful with ourselves, too much in awe of what might be wrong and what must be done to put us right.

HOW SHOULD I CARRY THINGS?

If you are faced with one large weight, redistribute it into two smaller, equal weights, carried in both hands, *tummy braced*. Do not let the weight pull you down, so that your tummy protrudes and shoulders droop. Make frequent stops. Carrying is a toil which must be taken seriously.

If the weight is a smaller more manageable size, then it is best carried, clutched to the chest. Never carry a weight out in front of the body. The leverage on the spine creates immense strain on your back.

Perhaps we should take a leaf out of the book of those living in the Indian subcontinent. The women carry objects on their heads, which totally eradicates any leverage problems, and the men carry large weights with poles over the shoulders, so the full brunt of the weight is carried by the ribcage. We are crazy to use our arms.

HOW CAN I COPE WITH LONG-DISTANCE TRAVEL?

Except for trains and planes with sleeping compartments, we have yet to invent a mass transportation system that does not involve sitting up. This is all very well if you want to read or write or take in the view, but it takes a heavy toll on the spine. Sitting makes the spine compress longitudinally – especially at the base – making it bunch down like a piano accordion, rarely getting a chance to elongate and 'suck in a deep breath'.

When you think about it, sitting is a very odd thing to do – folding up in the middle and perching the tail on a convenient surface. Spinally speaking, squatting is an ancient and much more suitable alternative. It demands the torso stay poised and alert rather than flopped and, apart from removing the ramming-up effect from below, the muscle effort dynamically decompresses the base of the spine. With squatting, we are kept aloft by the co-contraction of the paired tummy and back muscles. However, this is not the case with sitting: with a seat back for support, we flop. The abdominal wall relaxes as the girth slackens and the belly spills forward over the brim of the pelvis. The hydraulic sack qualities of the abdomen let go and the ribcage sags. This weighty collapse compresses not only the abdominal contents but also all the lumbar discs. The spine settles down into the pelvis and bleeds all the discs dry.

One of the earliest pieces of bio-mechanical research revealed that the pressure in the discs is highest when sitting and, as long as we remain there, the pressure continues. Relatively speaking, our discs dry out, with the greatest amount of fluid escaping in the first two hours. Like a sponge in a vice, water oozes out and is absorbed by the bloodstream. This loss of discoid fluid through vertical compression is known as 'axial creep'.

As more fluid squeezes out, like air out of a car tyre, the nucleus deflates and most weight is taken through the fibrous disc rim. The spine becomes brittle and cramped and is compromised in rebuffing impact from below, compression from above and jolts from the side. I believe this phenomenon is the chief background cause of human back pain. Even healthy spines can be made vulnerable by too much sitting – mainly because they are then so susceptible to injury. Furthermore, if a spine is riddled with stiff links, like the random scatter of rusty links in a bicycle chain, it is easy to see how long-term sitting can tickle up pre-existing problems as well. Sitting squeezes drier spots drier.

Provided that the disc has not irreversibly stiffened, most rehydration occurs spontaneously during sleep, as long as we are lying down. Each disc imbibes fluid and we actually 'grow' through the night as we undulate along the mattress. During the day we depend upon body movement to interrupt this shrinkage. Everyday activities such as bending, reaching, stretching, twisting, standing up and sitting down all exert a 'squash-release-suck' effect on the discs which pulls in water and boosts the spine's stature.

Sitting for long periods, say in an airline seat, brings together the two factors previously mentioned: the loss of fluid from the discs because of the raised intra-discal pressure, and the inability to recoup lost fluid because of the forced inactivity. Long-distance lorry drivers probably have the worst of it, with an incidence of back trouble four times the national average, probably triggered by heavy lifting between spells at the wheel.

A third phenomenon comes into play during extended periods of sitting and this relates to the squidgy nature of the tissues in and around the spine. The soft tissues of the spine are extremely vascular, that is, they have an abundant blood supply. The tissues themselves, ranging from the bone, disc, cartilage and capsule through to ligament and muscle, all have a high water content. You might say they are waterlogged, which, incidentally, explains why inflammation and its simultaneous swelling always cause such havoc, particularly in the back.

These fluids can be pushed into pooling pockets at the back of the spine if it remains kinked or bent over in one position for too long. In the case of a traveller sitting slumped for hours in a seat, or a carpenter crouched over a work bench all day, the front parts of the spinal joints are 'milked' as the fluids squeeze through to the back where things aren't so tight. Unfortunately, they then can't get back and become trapped as a bloated wedge of fluid. This accounts for the difficulty we all experience in standing upright again after long periods bent over – gardening or vacuuming or tinkering over a car engine. The collection of fluids on one side of the spine acts as a block to the spine realigning itself straight. This is known as 'creep in flexion'.

An acute back flare-up will often present like this, too. The sufferer stands bent forward and miserable and any attempt to straighten up will cause a searing pain as the legs crumble. Usually it is muscle spasm which has locked the spine crooked; pooling occurs but the pain will not ease until the spine has been gently straightened and the tissue fluids have rebalanced their distribution. The way to do this is described in Chapter 6 (see Figures 6.7.1 to 6.7.5).

A more common back condition is the older, drier back, which grumbles from time to time but really plays up during travel. The discs are dry and lacking in bounce. They are harder to squash flat and then puff up again and the back appears brittle and lacking in shock absorption. At the same time, all the other para-spinal tissues are drier, less elastic and less able to roll with the punches.

Or, you might be fit and young with just one level in a sleek and glistening spine behaving in this way because it has been damaged previously. This is one of the commonest conditions I see in clinical practice – an otherwise mobile and elastic spine, hampered by one stiff link in its midst. Even one segment misbehaving in this manner can cause the sort of 'old man's back' syndrome that is so often the source of much dismay. (You can see this in backs as young as 15 or 16 years old.)

It's obvious from all this that any back with a problem is going to be severely taxed by long-distance travel, whether it's a rusty spine or a solitary rusty link in a healthy spine. Hours of sitting sorely deprives it of its lubricating juices and you will often see people pulling themselves out of their seats and standing for a while, trying to coax their bent frames upright before they move off.

However, the good news with travelling is that although you cannot possibly avoid 'axial creep' – the slow settling of the spine down upon itself – you can avoid 'creep in flexion' by at least attempting to sit properly. If you avoid slumping in a heavy and hopeless C-shaped curve, you will minimise the bentness. Keeping your seat-belt on also helps because it stops your bottom sliding forward on the seat and prevents your shoulders slumping.

Another adverse effect of travel comes from prolonged vibration. Vibration speeds up the loss of fluid from the discs. Air travellers may fare better than those in trains or cars simply because the vibration is less, however, there are other problems with planes, not least the longer hours, cramped conditions and reduced cabin pressure. Although the plane may be flying at an altitude of 9,000 metres, cabin pressure is maintained at a level of 2,000 metres. This is considerably less than the air pressure at sea level and is another reason why our feet swell.

There are a few things you can do, and, with the inertia, vibration, settling and looping of a travelling spine, it certainly needs some help.

Some of them you will do instinctively anyway, like arching in the seat and stretching the arms in a subconscious attempt to disimpact and reflate the spine. But sometimes you'll see passengers disregard the signals and straightaway haul themselves out of their seat, only to find that their backs won't straighten. Then they compound the damage by reaching up to get baggage out of the overhead lockers.

I have treated many a back that has come to grief at this point. A spine that is not only compressed but also set lopsided in a semi-rigid hoop, is hardly in a condition to extend itself upwards in one jerk, not to mention saddle itself with a barrage of baggage coming down from above. And the straw that breaks the passenger's back, so to speak, comes at the baggage claim. Big bags create real mischief. Usually they are so heavy that they can only be carried one at a time, and the real killer is yanking them off the moving track.

You can minimise the ructions by following a few simple precautions. Needless to say, they all revolve around *movement*. Basically, the more you move, the better – though not at the expense of your fellow passengers' comfort. Don't wriggle around in your seat and be a nuisance in the aisles, squatting and touching your toes. There are other things you can do while sitting in your seat that are also effective.

The most important thing is your long-term sitting position: try to keep a hollowing arch in your lumbar spine – never allow it to slump in a broad 'C'. Keep your bottom as close as possible to the seat-back, because the further it slides forward, the further it takes your lower back away from support and the more you flop. Stuff a small airline pillow into the transitional area of your spine (see 'Which is the Best Chair?', Chapter 9) to stop your spine creeping vertically down the back of the seat. Apart from neck support, this is the most effective way to use these pillows. However, most people position them too low and end up almost sitting on them. Keep monitoring your position and if you find yourself creeping forward, shift backwards again. 'Walk' backwards on your buttocks to get to the back of the seat, or lever yourself back by using the arm-rests. Both actions dramatically alter the pressure in your discs and check the spine's impaction.

The slowing of the circulation, in particular the venous return of blood up from the legs to the heart, is another consequence of lengthy air travel, and it's an uphill job keeping it working efficiently. This is partly due to reduced cabin pressure, which facilitates the pooling of blood in the lower legs, and partly due to cramped inactivity. Another impediment is the kinking of the large veins of the pelvis as they traverse the front of the hip joints. The angled hips obstruct the flow of blood and create back-pressure in the venous system; sitting with your legs crossed only adds to this. A fourth impediment to circulation is the sitting pressure on the buttocks and backs of the thighs which blocks the passage of blood through the tissues. The recent interest in cases of deep vein thrombosis is some indication of the numbers of airline passengers who have suffered the final insult of veins in the leg clogging and forming clots.

This is a major nursing hazard in caring for the incapacitated and the elderly. Deprived of a healthy flow of blood, the veins in the leg can clot or the tissues quickly break down and 'bedsores' develop from the pressure of body weight. Although travellers are not prone to such extremes, the process is the same: blood flow is hampered when passing through pressure areas.

To help your joints, circulation, digestion and peace of mind while travelling, you need movement.

Probably the most effective means of restoring juice to the lower discs is to simply rock your spine back and forth as you sit there. You can do it in two ways. The first is by humping and hollowing the lumbar spine in and out of a concave and convex attitude. The more exaggerated the movement the better: imagine, as you rock over the discs, that you are activating them like a vertical row of mini-bellows, sucking fluid in and out. Emphasise the concave phase to counter all those hours spent slumped. Do this by thrusting your fists into the small of your back to reinforce the forward movement. Push forward three times for every hump backwards.

The other way to open and close the discs is by a sideways movement, although the available freedom in this direction is much less. Rock from one buttock to the other, at the same time bending your trunk sideways as you lift your weight off the seat. This exercise requires a good deal of tummy strength and incidentally is very effective in shrinking the waistline.

These two exercises help to 'prime' the discs in readiness for more adventurous tasks, like wrestling with the baggage. But another standby is a sitting version of the exercise shown in Chapter 6, Figure 6.9.1. In a semi-recumbent position, bring both thighs up onto your chest, crossing your ankles (if there is room) and bounce them gently with both hands.

(Impossible in a skirt!) Repeat the procedure many times; you cannot overdo it.

You can also exercise the calves and lower legs to reduce swollen feet. Sit squarely in the seat with your legs bent at an obtuse angle and feet planted firmly on the floor. Lift both heels and point your toes, then reverse the action. Press both heels into the floor and pull your toes back as far as they will go. Repeat over and over again for as long as you can endure before cramp creeps in.

This reduces the swelling through an alternate pumping action of the muscles at the front and back of the shins. When a muscle contracts, its fibres shorten and its bulk thickens, pressing against the casing of the skin of the lower leg. This pumps the interstitial fluids back into the circulation towards the heart. This 'muscle pump' operates all the time, assisting the heart in shunting the circulation around the body. Easy to see why gentle activity helps with cardiac problems.

Finally, when you stand up, be careful. You have been impacting a long time. Use your thigh muscles to push you up and remember to brace your stomach. If you have only partially unkinked your spine with the humping and hollowing exercise, you will need to do a bit more once you are upright. Push your hands into your back and prise yourself straight. Then arch backwards a few times, especially before you start carrying heavy bags.

9 Your Other Questions Answered

With an estimated nine out of ten in the population at some stage suffering backache, you can be sure that, no matter how miserable you are, you are not alone.

From my experience in handling all kinds of backs, the following are the commonest questions asked. I have presented them to you as they are presented to me.

WHAT IS GOOD POSTURE?

Good posture is the best way for the skeleton to hold itself to carry the body's weight easily. This means that in practice, from the side view, your centre of gravity passes in a straight line through the ear, the tip of the shoulder, the centre of the fourth lumbar vertebra, slightly in front of the knee and just behind the ankle-bone of the foot.

Pronounced abnormalities of posture cause the mechanics of the spine, limbs and head to be more laboured. The weight of the body is not well managed so the stresses of additional daily toil are not easily tolerated. Poor low back posture has direct ramifications for the breakdown of the front or back compartments of the spine.

Faulty posture over a long period will chronically strain the skeleton and ultimately cause pain.

The three main anomalies of posture are:

1. An increased lumbar lordosis or hollowed low back. This is often combined with short hip flexors, which make the front of the hips tight so that you have to take shorter steps.
2. The lumbar kyphosis or humped low back. This may be associated with a round-shouldered hunch and a sunken abdomen with a transverse crease at waist level. It also goes with tight hamstrings.
3. The 'too straight back' where there is insufficient thoracic curve. This is often associated with a 'poke' neck.

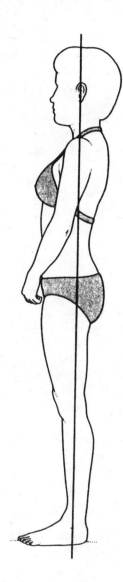

Figure 9.1 Ideal posture.

Changing a bad posture is never easy. It is, after all, a habit of a lifetime. Posture is also intimately related to psychological factors and therefore unlikely to be corrected by physical measures alone. However, if bad posture can be improved, it makes the world of difference to your back – not to mention your feelings of well-being.

With bad posture, the best approach is manual mobilisation of any stiff segments – so the spine is free to shuffle about internally to assume a better stance – and then stretching and strengthening exercises where structures are tight and weak.

Here are the main stretching and strengthening exercises to counteract the common postural faults.

(1) The Too Hollow Low Back

An optimal lumbar hollow helps us ride out impact. It lets the spine sink and spring as the foot strikes the ground with each step. Just the right amount of lordosis allows the lumbar segments to squelch forward slightly as the back takes weight. (You see this beautifully with the long-distance African runners.) The mechanism is kept in trim by the 'anterior longitudinal ligament', which is like a strong elastic tape down the front of the vertebral bodies that prevents them splaying open too far. Too much lordosis reduces the bounce in the low back and causes excessive weight to be taken through the facets at the *back* of the spine.

The best technique for restoring lumbar bounce involves using the BackBlock. It not only separates the segments but stretches the tight structures at the front of the hips which keep the front of the pelvis permanently tipped forward. Another way of stretching tight hip flexors individually is to pull one knee up at a time and bounce it hard on the chest while leaving the other leg hanging off the side edge of the bed (Figure 6.16, Chapter 6). Bouncing the knees to the chest (in the lying position) and toe touching (in the standing position) complement the BackBlock in stretching all those tight structures down the *back* of the spine.

To strengthen a loose tummy that is not providing adequate retaining-wall support for your spine, you need to do plenty of sit-ups daily – more than the thirty incorporated with the BackBlock regime. To help realign the tipped-forward pelvis, you will also need to strengthen the gluteal muscles. The best way to do this is by pelvic bridging exercises; lying on your back with the knees crooked, lifting your bottom off the floor and making a clean line between your knees and shoulders.

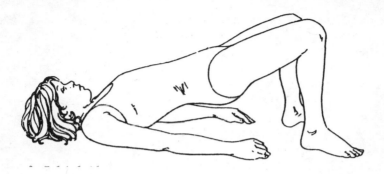

Figure 9.2 Pelvic bridging increases the strength of the muscles of the buttocks. Their added strength helps to reduce excessive lumbar hollowing.

(2) The Too Round Back

When a spine bears weight through a too-rounded lower back its ability to accept shock is compromised. Denied a natural bowing forward of the segments on impact, most weight is therefore taken through the neuro-central core through the disc-vertebra mechanisms. Because the facets are pulled apart and open in the kyphosed position, no weight is taken through the back of the spine. Thus a kyphosed posture speeds up breakdown of low lumbar discs.

Using a BackBlock is the best way to re-establish a lumbar lordosis, too. Almost certainly, you will also need to use it under the upper back to un-hunch the shoulders. You can increase the stretch by lying prone on the floor with a pile of pillows under your ribcage. As you relax, the lumbar spine will sink deeper into an arch, totally unlike its habitual forward slump. You can progress it by pushing up on extended arms to arch the spine backwards (see Figure 6.7.4, Chapter 6).

In the absence of a BackBlock (some people make do with a 7cm pile of books), you can stretch a hunched thorax by lying backwards off the edge of a bed (with the edge of the mattress under the apex of the curve of the thorax). In this position, bounce the arms back over your head in a gentle, oscillatory way to gently stretch out the pectoral area. Keep the elbows straight and arms close to the ears.

To strengthen the muscles that hold you up straight, lie face down on the floor with two pillows under your belly. With both hands behind your head,

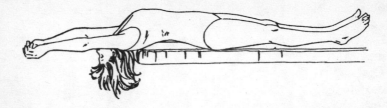

Figure 9.3 The thorax stretch to 'undo' habitual working postures.

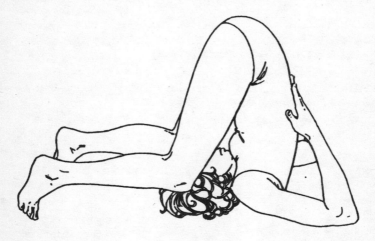

Figure 9.4 By stretching the spine, particularly between the shoulder blades, the 'Plough' helps rectify a poke neck.

lift the head and legs off the floor. This particularly works the 'long back extensors' and helps to hold the spine erect (see Figure 6.20, Chapter 6).

(3) The Too-Straight Back

Both the above sets of exercises will help here, but the emphasis should be on loosening rather than on strengthening. The only way to deal with a 'poke' neck is by restoring more roundness to the thoracic area. So although, on face value, the following procedure appears to push your neck forward more, it actually deals with the problem at source. You must lie flat on your back on the floor and swing your legs up over your head, resting your toes on the floor behind you. In yoga this is called the 'Plough' and it is a wonderful experience for the entire spine. The exercise can be progressed by lowering your legs down astride your head to rest your knees beside the ears. NOTE: The neck must be protected by placing several layers of folded towel under the prominent bone at the base of your neck.

This exercise is always difficult and must be done very gently to start with. It may be months before you can get the knees on the floor beside the ears. Take it easy!

WHY IS LYING DOWN SO UNCOMFORTABLE?

If lying down is painful, it is probably what you are lying on! A soft bed is usually the culprit (see 'What Is the Best Bed?' next section). By and large, lying down is the most comfortable position for a painful back: it is in repose, relieved of postural and gravitational stresses, so it is more likely to relax. The intra-discal pressure is then at its lowest and the spine actually elongates this way during sleep.

Spinal lengthening comes about for two reasons: first, the natural curves of the spine which have increased through the day, weighed down by tiredness and hard work, flatten out again in the horizontal position. Secondly, the discs actually suck in fluid when relieved of weight-bearing pressures. This expands the discs and lengthens the spine.

During the day, there is a net flow of fluid out of the discs. As they squash down, the spine imperceptibly settles down upon itself and becomes more brittle – especially after lengthy periods of sitting or standing. That's when we feel an irresistible desire to stretch and bend the body to puff up the discs and make ourselves more comfortable again.

All this being so, back problems rarely worsen with lying down. However, there are exceptions.

In cases of multiple disc degeneration, there will be discomfort after lying and the back will be especially stiff in the mornings. This may be because the mesh of the disc walls is so unstretchable, it cannot pull apart to allow the nucleus to imbibe fluid. Any increase in disc volume is met with an increased tension in the disc walls, making the low back very stiff and painful first thing. Getting up and moving about stirs the segments out of their torpor and eases the pain, but it may take an hour or two before you get going.

With these backs, a large part of treatment involves stretching the meshed disc walls. This is initially done by using the BackBlock and all-round spinal stretching, although diagonal twisting exercises particularly target the disc walls (see The Floor Twist, pages 121–2) and make the spine loosen up more quickly.

Another reason for pain after lying is that muscles in spasm often get stiffer. Muscles automatically go into protective mode to save a sore joint being pulled about. Problems worsen when spasming muscles prevent too much movement and make the joint more rigid. To break this cycle you must stretch the muscles to release their hold. (When you are in less pain you can also switch them off physiologically by doing hard tummy exercises – curl-ups.)

In the meantime, to loosen yourself in the mornings, you should always do the rocking knees exercise on waking. Lie on your back and gently bring one knee to the chest. Pull it up and release it in small, oscillatory movements, repeating it many times. Then do the same with the other leg. It is often not manageable lifting both legs together. They are too heavy and it isn't easy keeping a relaxing rhythm going. After this has loosened you up a bit, you can get down on to the floor and do spinal rolling (see Chapter 6).

All backs, except those kept habitually in a rounded slump, are strained by sleeping face down. This is because the lumbar spine lies slung between two supports, the ribcage and the pelvis. With the relaxation induced by sleep, the lumbar spine quietly sags into a deep hollow. This is fine if all the joints are healthy and elastic but, if not, it will get hurt all over again. Lying prone particularly targets a facet joint problem because the spine hangs on these joints; the weight of the sagging spine tugs at the unstretchable link. As a consequence, you wake set rigid in the low back, making it very difficult to get up.

WHAT IS THE BEST BED?

I always find this a difficult question to answer, because it depends on two variables: your weight (and your partner's weight) and your degree of stiffness. There is always debate over whether beds should allow your spine to hollow or not.

Bear in mind that we change our sleep position hundreds of times a night, so that any one position is of no particular relevance because we so quickly move out of it. So, don't worry what a bed does, or does not do, to the various pathologies. The important thing is that your bed *prevents you lapsing into extremes of posture*. The spine needs support, firm support, to maintain, as nearly as possible, its natural curves. This helps it relax and grow along the mattress overnight so that your discs are puffed up and buoyant by morning.

A soft, sagging mattress keeps the spine bunched in, which brings on pain by allowing the spine to sag. The stiff joints cannot give, so they sag and are strained in the process. You then wake up stiff because the muscles have gone into protective spasm and you are stuck; rather like a beetle stranded on its back, you have to roll over and lever yourself up sideways to get out of bed. Getting socks on is out of the question.

Just to confuse things, sleeping on a firm mattress is not always comfortable, either! All too often, fed up with having back pain and heeding the advice of thousands of well-meaning friends, you go out and spend a small fortune on the latest orthopaedic bed, only to find when you get it home that it is impossible to sleep on. As a general rule, the stiffer the spine, the less able it is to adapt to a very hard bed. If you are extremely stiff at every spinal level, then you will be better in the interim, before your spine has been made supple again, sleeping on a medium-hard mattress. At least there is some contour support rather than the two unresilient obstacles, the spine and the mattress, fighting it out till dawn.

As a general rule, the ideal bed should comfortably take your weight as you sit on the edge of it and should feel firmly springy. The more healthy and elastic the spine, the more support it needs in sleep and therefore the harder the mattress should be.

IN WHICH POSITION SHOULD I SLEEP?

Sleep in any position that is comfortable.

Backs with an increased lumbar hollow are uncomfortable lying face down because the hollow increases. On the other hand, if you have a rounded low back, you may enjoy lying this way because it straightens you out. If you are in the middle of a nasty back flare-up, the most comfortable position is on your side cuddling a pillow, with another between your knees, both knees drawn up.

Another comfortable position, especially if you have just done something to your back (see 'Have I Put My Back Out?' Chapter 3), is lying on the floor with both calves supported, hips at ninety degrees. If the support surface is too low, build it up with cushions so the bottom is lifted slightly off the floor. The effect of this is twofold. First, it puts the lumbar spine in its most neutral position, which reduces the pressure between the segments and prevents muscle spasm taking hold. And secondly, lifting the back off the floor gives the spine gentle traction, which separates the jammed joint.

Before getting up from this position, gently tilt, swivel and roll the pelvis. This presses the jammed segment into the floor and helps loosen it.

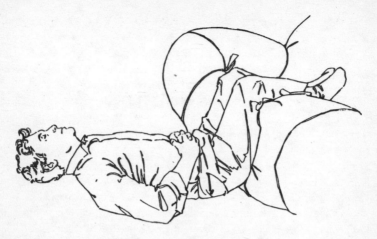

Figure 9.5 An excellent position for relieving an acutely painful back.

WHY IS SITTING SO UNCOMFORTABLE?

Although providing recuperation for aching feet and legs, sitting is not good for backs. The intra-discal pressure with sitting is much greater than standing or lying. Fluid leaches from the lowermost discs, making the base of the spine impacted and brittle. This creates the pre-pathology for more serious back problems to develop.

The variation on this theme is the back that is fine while sitting but gives an excruciating jab of pain as you go to stand up.

There are two theories about what is going on here.

The first is the puffy wedge of fluid that collects in the back compartments of the spine when it stays hooped forward, even more so at an inflamed level. The back literally 'pinches' these bloated structures when it tries to jack itself straight. Pain on rising from sitting also indicates 'segmental instability' caused by one weak link in the spine. When the spine tips forward to get up, there is a shearing strain across the lumbar segments. The weaker segment goes to slip forward, out of the column, and there is a sharp pain as the muscles grab it.

In both cases, pain can be minimised by bracing the tummy before rising. This reduces the forward inclination of the spine and raises the intra-abdominal pressure. It enhances the tummy's role as a hydraulic sack, thus exerting back pressure on the spine to prevent the vertebrae slipping forward. You can then rise by using the powerful muscles of the thighs, rather than by lurching forward so that the centre of gravity is over your feet.

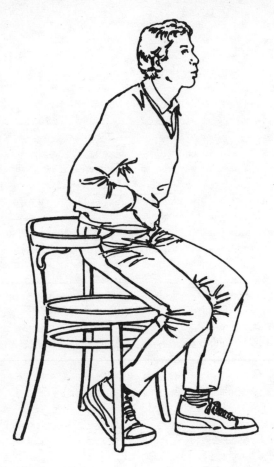

Figure 9.6 The best way to rise from a seat is to brace the abdomen with a firm, restraining hand and use the thighs to elevate the body.

The other state of affairs that makes sitting uncomfortable is a bit more complicated, though it only strikes when you have been sitting for some time.

Sometimes, as a result of severe inflammation of one of the spinal joints, all the soft-tissue structures nearby (except the bone itself) are affected by the process. The dura, the loose membranous sack that wraps around the spinal cord, may also be included in the inflammatory process.

All the different tissues ooze clear lymph fluid as a result of the inflammation. But, because you are in too much pain to move, this fluid gradually becomes gluey and sticky as it pools, instead of being pumped away in the course of normal activity. Eventually the stagnant fluid transforms into 'adhesions' (a stringy mass of junk), which then tether the delicate dural membrane to the inside wall of the spinal canal.

After the acute back pain has passed and you are up and about, this dural tethering is barely noticeable. Indeed, activities that do not stretch the spine will not provoke pain from the harnessed dura. However, with prolonged sitting, the spine tends to slump deeper as you get more tired and heavy. As the back bows more deeply, the spine increases in length and the cord inside the canal stretches tight. This has the effect of drawing the cord in from the side-walls of the vertebral canal, thus also drawing the spinal nerves back in through their exit-canals.

The actual dural tethering is brought about by many hair-like strands of adhesions binding the dura to the wall of the spinal canal, rather like the hairs on Gulliver's head being pegged to the ground by the Lilliputians! Because the dura cannot stretch as the spine elongates, it gets tugged and therefore inflamed. Common signs of dural tethering are back and/or leg pain after lengthy periods of sitting, typically after long car or aeroplane journeys.

The only way to treat this problem is to use the same treatment principles applied in treating all other problems of inelasticity of soft tissues – gentle stretching to regain normal stretchability.

The way to do this is to bend the body in two at waist level, either by bringing the head to the knees while standing (see Figure 6.11.2, Chapter 6), or swinging the bad leg forward in repeated straight-leg high kicks.

With the head-to-knee exercise, the forward movement of the head tends to pull the cord 'upwards' inside the spinal canal thus freeing it. On the other hand, the leg-kicks pull the spinal cord 'downwards' in the spinal canal, freeing it in that direction.

When both exercises have become relatively pain free, they should be tried in combination. Stand on the good leg with the bad leg supported on a low stool and the knee as straight as possible. Gently force the head towards the knee of the supported leg while gently bouncing the tight knee downwards until the tightness eases.

As this becomes less painful, either raise the supporting surface for the bad leg or start the exercise with the bad leg supported on a low chair and progress to supporting it on the kitchen table. The process is gradual and must not be hurried. Nervous tissue and its protective covering do not tolerate stampeding tactics!

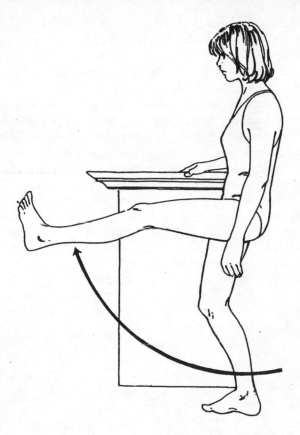

Figure 9.7 Straight-leg kicking is the most effective means of freeing a tethered nerve root.

WHICH IS THE BEST CHAIR?

A good chair is one which maintains a proper lumbar lordosis.

When you sit, your spine is stacked upright upon itself, supporting its weight against gravity. A little support in the right place makes all the difference between a comfortable chair and a dreadful one.

Sitting becomes uncomfortable when chairs allow the spine to adopt extremes of posture, although they more commonly encourage slumping than hollowing. Both facet joint problems and dry, thinning discs – the two most common causes of pain from the back – are aggravated by bad chairs.

In the case of facet trouble, the joints complain when they are pulled apart and kept open by the back sitting in a hooped slump. The 'C' position tugs at the fibrosed facet capsules and causes a sharp, bilateral pain, which spreads out wide of the spine. This sort of pain is relieved by over-arching backwards and digging the fingers in deep beside the spine. Pressure here often gives a 'sweet pain', which is shrill but brings relief.

Degenerated discs are also uncomfortable when posture is stooped because it forces all the weight of the upper body down through the neurocentral core (the disc-vertebra part of the spine). This type of back problem can be greatly relieved by using a chair that encourages a better lordosis. This offloads some of the compression onto the facets and is best achieved, in the first instance, by tipping the front of the seat down a few degrees.

The following is a brief run-down on what makes a good or bad chair.

The worst chair is one with a completely straight back at right angles to a completely straight seat; sitting on one of these for any length of time can be purgatory! The rounded, more protuberant part of the spine (the thoracic kyphosis) is unable to arch back naturally over the lumbar spine because the straight chair-back is in the way. The whole upper body area is therefore pushed forward, in front of the line of gravity, making the low back slump and the muscles work overtime to stop the upper body crumpling completely forward. After a while, the muscles start to fatigue and a twingeing ache sets in.

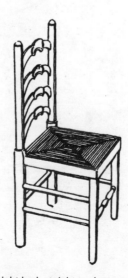

Figure 9.8 The worst chair – a straight back at right angles to a straight seat.

If the spine is not able to carry itself in a balanced equilibrium, with just as much weight sitting behind the line of gravity as in front, it will ache, even if the back is usually healthy. How awful to sit in a chair that makes even a healthy back ache! And there are plenty of them about, usually in restaurants. The only way to get comfortable on one of these fiendish chairs is to perch one's bottom right on the front edge of the seat and recline back, so that only the transitional curve of the spine (that area between lumbar hollow and the thoracic hump) rests against the chair. However, it is a very inelegant, crumpled way of sitting and impossible to maintain for too long.

A chair-back that slopes backwards a few degrees beyond the vertical, so that it lies in line with the transitional curve as it sweeps up from the lumbar region, is much more comfortable. It is quite astonishing how this alteration in design can make such a difference.

A particularly bad type of chair often has a straw base, which slopes down in the centre of the seat so that the front edge of the chair frame neatly cuts into the back of the thighs in a most uncomfortable manner. The only way to relieve the pressure is to either cross the legs, which is bad for spinal alignment (and terrible for varicose veins), or hook the heels over the chair-rungs at the front of the chair, which also does terrible things to the posture.

The best type of functional all-purpose chair is the transitional bar-support chair. These are commonly regarded as typists' chairs and are ideal

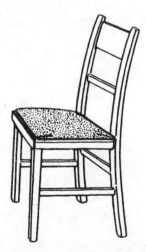

Figure 9.9 A better chair – the back slopes backwards a few degrees.

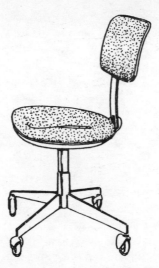

Figure 9.10 The typist's chair with the upholstered pad which nudges into the high lumbar/low thoracic spine (the transitional curve).

where the occupant does not need to lean forward to work. The back-support section of these chairs consists of a soft but firm upholstered pad which nudges transversely across the spine, just under the lower ribs at the back. If this transverse pad is connected to a hinge, the arrangement is even better. It not only allows the occupant the freedom to arch backwards to stretch after periods of concentration, but its variable backwards angulation allows the spine to rest on the soft pad and off-load some of its weight.

The back support, contoured to the transitional curve, helps to lift the spine as it passes back over the centre of gravity. Due to the partial unloading of the heavy weight of the torso, the lumbar spine hangs better below the support, in a much more pleasing alignment.

There is a satisfactory variation of the typist's chair manufactured as a dining-chair. This has a back support that encircles the body at lower-rib level, continuing around the sides as arm supports. If the chair is well padded it helps, as does a slight bevelling of the chair-back where it comes in contact with the spine. Unfortunately, most chairs of the transitional-bar design fail to extend high enough and therefore rarely offer proper support.

Excellent though typists' chairs are, they are a bit insubstantial. You won't find top executives using them behind their expansive desks; they want a chair to match their desk. The bulky, uncontoured chair of the

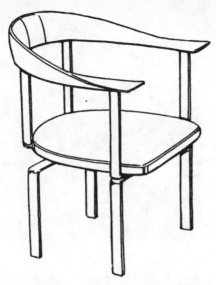

Figure 9.11 The dining-chair with its back support encircling the body at lower rib level.

highly stuffed variety is commonly seen here, and they are bad for backs. They are usually old-fashioned, with a well-padded, gently sloping back support rising from a well-sprung seat that is far too deep. They often have bulky arm-rests, which is the best thing about them – they are placed at exactly the right height to take weight through the arms. Upholstered chair arms are essential if you are going to spend time in a chair, because they can bear almost a quarter of body weight (22 per cent).

The common fault with bulky chairs is that their seat is too deep to support the low back. Despite the 'grand' design you will rather ingloriously have to support your back with pillows to prevent your low back slumping into a 'C'.

It's worth noting that ergonomically designed chairs are often not good enough, and although some are better than others, all are expensive. The better ones are adjustable everywhere to suit people of all shapes and sizes. In particular, they must have a lever to alter the angle of the seat, allowing it to be dipped down at the front (the degree depending on how readily the spine slumps). Chairs should also be adjustable in height, so that with the feet flat on the floor your knees are just below hip-level. Any lower and the back will over-arch; any higher and the spine will hump.

The back support should exaggerate a lumbar hollow, preferably with a

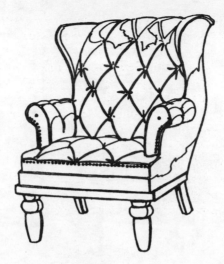

Figure 9.12 The bulky, uncontoured chair.

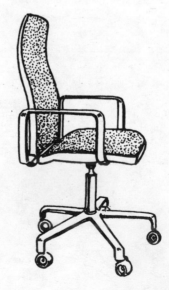

Figure 9.13 Well-contoured chairs have a softly contoured protuberance that extends well up the spine. However, most contoured chairs conform too readily to the non-tired shape of the occupant.

firm, upholstered pad that makes good contact with the spine, well up into the transitional curve area. If it is ample enough, this pad will 'lift' the upper body, as discussed earlier. There is no real need to support the spine beyond the transitional curve. Head-rests are usually a nuisance.

An ordinary bulky chair such as the one described earlier is infinitely preferable to poorly contoured ergonomic chairs. Badly contoured chairs conform too readily to the non-tired posture of the occupant and thus fail to provide adequate support. They don't sufficiently over-accentuate good spinal alignment. They fail to lift and support the heavy chest and head, and they often have a too deep thoracic curve so that unless you are a man with a great barrel chest, you are swallowed up in the hollow – especially if the protruding neck-pad is too high, which it often is. The old economy-class aircraft seats were often badly contoured, but aircraft seats are steadily improving.

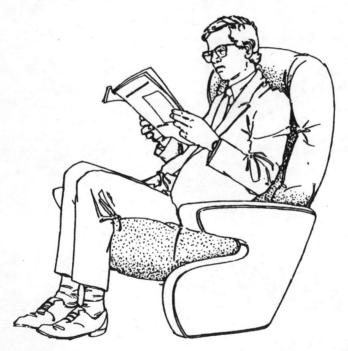

Figure 9.14 The old-fashioned average economy-class aircraft seat provides no support for a sitting spine.

The soft, squashy and deep chair or sofa that allows the whole spine to collapse in one continues 'C' bend needs mentioning here because it is so bad for your back. You are better off lying on the floor over your BackBlock. Usually made entirely of foam, with no proper base, this type of furniture typically causes an ache in the low back, even in healthy individuals, because it allows the spine to bear weight in such a grotesque way. By allowing the spine to adopt a slumped position, the vertebrae pinch together at the front and gape open at the back so that when you get up, you can hardly straighten. You are thus forced to move about for a minute or two fully bent forward, and have to push your hands into the small of your back to push yourself straight.

Here are a couple of rules on good seating:

1. The seat part must not be too deep. If it is, it will be impossible to sit back comfortably, with the low back properly supported and the feet resting squarely on the floor. In extreme cases, the front edge of the seat will press into the back of the calves, and the feet will barely reach the floor. The low back then sags into a deep, uncomfortable curve because there is no back support to hold it upright.

2. The optimum height of a chair seat above the floor should place the knees just slightly lower than the hips. If the chair is any lower, forcing the knees higher, the low back will slump into a 'C'. It will also take too much effort to get out of it. If the seat is too high, so the knees are substantially lower than the hips – and particularly if the feet cannot even reach the floor – you will be very uncomfortable indeed. That's why many public bars have floor

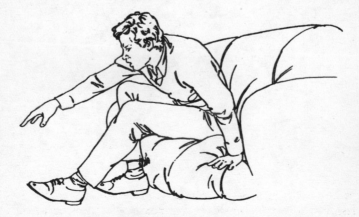

Figure 9.15 The soft-foam sofa; impossible to sit in and impossible to get out of.

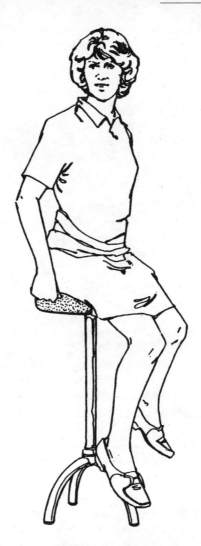

Figure 9.16 Two heavily hanging legs pull the lumbar spine forward in to an uncomfortable arch.

rails to make their patrons more comfortable during extended drinking sessions. Cocking one foot up prevents the low back sagging, whether you are sitting on a stool or standing up at the bar.

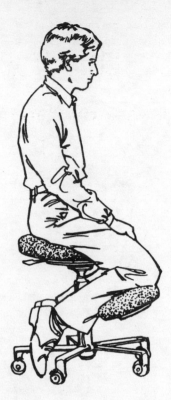

Figure 9.17 The ingenious Balans chair.

My favourite chair is the 'Balans' chair, made originally in Scandinavia. These are cleverly designed so the legs bear weight as well as the sitting bones. The small, forward-angled seat tips the pelvis forward, which achieves two things: it decreases the pressure on the buttocks, so the spine avoids direct compression, and it allows weight to be taken through the knees. Substantial pressure is taken through bulky, upholstered knee pads, which nestle into the housemaid's bump below the kneecaps. The main advantage of this chair is that it makes the spine automatically assume the perfect 'S' alignment, much in the same way as when riding or a horse or squatting. (Just try squatting for a bit. You will quickly see how pleasingly the spine hangs.)

There are two disadvantages of the Balans chair. First, it encourages the lumbar spine to hollow forward, and for backs that already exhibit too much scoop, sitting will be painful. This can be partly minimised by lowering the seat, thus putting the bottom almost on the heels. And while the heels do not actually take weight, it can be a strain on the ankles, not to mention the knees – this, of course, is the second disadvantage of this type of chair.

WHY IS STANDING SO UNCOMFORTABLE?

Standing tends to accentuate bad postures. It allows the spine to steadily deflate and compress its lower segments. Although you may have pain when standing around or casually sauntering, you may be completely free of it while bustling about with great purpose. This is because greater activity demands better postural control, with all the muscles working harder. The trimmer tummy keeps the spine taut and aloft, with a minimum of pressure on its base.

There is another specific condition where back pain is much worse when standing. It is associated with an overwhelming desire to sit down to relieve pain. It is called spondylolisthesis – the slipping forward of one vertebra (and the spine above it) off the front of the vertebra below. It happens when the bony hooks at the back (which are in fact the facet joints) are broken or otherwise made incompetent. They then fail to hold the spine in place.

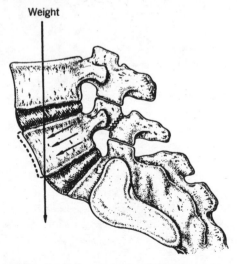

Figure 9.18 Spondylolisthesis, where the natural bony hook at the back of a segment becomes incompetent and fails to prevent the vertebra slipping forward.

Spondylolisthesis commonly occurs at the two lowest lumbar levels: L5 slipping off the sacrum, or L4 off L5. The incidence of slip is higher here because the hollowing of lordosis is greater and the vertebrae sit at a steeper angle. A lumbar lordosis is more pronounced with standing, but as the pelvis tips back when sitting, it almost disappears. Thus, standing increases the shearing strain across the low segments. The increased pain is caused by the slip stretching the soft tissues which are trying to keep everything in place.

The treatment of serious spondylolisthesis is surgical fusion of the slipping level, especially if there is severe pain, and even more especially if the slip is increasing.

If symptoms are not marked, spondylolistheses do well with manual mobilisation of the levels above and below the slip (which have usually become stiff as a compensatory development), followed by the intrinsic spinal stabilising exercises to bind the weak link together again (see Figures 6.25.1 to 6.25.3, Chapter 6). In some cases of quite marked slip – of a centimetre or so – there may be no symptoms at all. You may go through life never even knowing you had it.

IS SEX BAD FOR MY BACK?

I have always had a feeling that patients who ask me this question secretly hope that I will throw up my hands in horror and forbid all forms of sexual activity under pain of death. I sense they want me to excuse them from the travails of the bedroom.

Truth is, a little gentle sex is about the best thing you can do for a back – especially if you are on top. But if the act is too aggressive, with lots of heavy banging around, then you will inevitably thump yours and your partner's spine around.

It is perhaps a clever trick of nature that the muscles used during coitus are the very same ones that hold us upright and propel us forward; the two fundamentals of existence – being upright and getting about. Believe it or not, sex comes third!

The first muscle group is the strong gluteals – the buttocks – perhaps the strongest group in the body. They are in action every moment we are upright; a low-grade contraction keeps us from folding up at the hips. They also thrust the body forward on the weight-bearing leg in the support phase of walking.

The second muscle group is the abdominals – the tummy muscles – which, fortunately for most of us, can get away with not being as strong as they might. Their primary role is holding the belly in to act as a brace, thus preventing the spine from protruding forward at low lumbar level. Their lesser role is the pelvic rolling action, bringing it from the hollow-backed position to the humped-back position.

The best action for both partners during intercourse is gentle, rhythmic rolling of the pelvis where the spine humps and hollows alternately. The pelvic action is supplied by the tummy muscles and the thrusting action by the gluteals. Voilá! (Strictly speaking, anybody who has a slack tummy is sure to be a lousy lover. You'd better take a look at yours.)

IS HOUSEWORK BAD FOR MY BACK?

The problem with housework is that it is exacting and tiring without being sufficiently energetic. It involves long periods of toiling at awkward angles, usually with the shoulders stooped and the head bowed, but the whole activity is not dynamic enough to benefit the skeleton.

Modern gadgetry has made things easier but not easy enough. The gutsy stuff has been taken out so we are left with the paltry limited-range activity so commonplace in our modern lives. We are not kept fit; just worn down.

In the pursuit of a rationale to account for non-specific aches and pains from people involved in tedious (and repetitive) manual work, a modern syndrome has evolved. Its name: repetitive strain injury (RSI).

If you think about it rationally, it is hardly surprising that, in some instances, the skeleton makes known its objection to the uses we put it to. It is another consequence of the machine-dominated world in which we live.

Small, repetitive movements create enormous wear and tear on the joints. Imagine the people who stand at production lines and repeat the same movement, day in day out; or better still, a computer operator spending hour upon hour focusing the whole body on the winking movement of one small cursor. The limited range of movement, as well as the lack of variety, causes trouble; the repetition is another thing. If our movements involved more flourish and flamboyance our postures would not be so static and more blood supply would be called in to lubricate the working parts.

As it is, the spine becomes congealed into a semi-rigid pole and the joints become locked in meagre activity patterns. The tendons of the arms start to chafe and fray, like the fibres of old rope working back and forth around a pulley. Of course, if you then add to this the complete picture of lethargic leisure hours, with too many cigarettes and cups of coffee, then aches and pains are a foregone conclusion.

Three types of housework spring to mind as being the most demanding on the human frame: vacuum cleaning, ironing and making beds.

Vacuuming is a problem, especially if the machine is one that you pull along the floor behind you. It forces you to work bent over, pushing the nozzle across the floor, and we all know that sustained bending is bad, as is pushing (see 'What is Wrong With Pushing?' Chapter 8).

However, reducing the suction makes it easier to push the head across the carpet. It also helps if you push the head away with the nozzle at an angle that prevents it from sucking, then flatten it on to the floor as you pull it back, so it works as you pull it towards you. Try making the rigid tubing as long as possible so you can push from hip height. And try to keep as upright as possible as you work, *keeping the tummy braced*.

The old-fashioned upright cleaners are better for backs than the cylindrical ones because they have a different action. They have a circular rotating brush, which beats the carpet to get the dust airborne, then sucks it up. This, together with the fact that the head runs on wheels, means it is much easier to push. These machines are also easier because they allow you to stand more upright. However, they are not as good for getting into corners and under beds.

Ironing is a problem, too, because it involves such laboured hours spent standing still. Inevitably, the spine sinks into deeper and deeper curves as the tummy gradually gives up the battle of keeping the spine in trim. My advice is either to iron while sitting on a shooting stick or put a small box on the floor to elevate one foot. The box should be quite robust so it actually takes your weight, rather like the foot-rail in the public bar, and also takes the sag out of your low back by rolling the pelvis back. It makes long ironing sessions so much easier.

Making beds is also a problem, especially low double beds. It is not so much the bending as lifting up the mattress and tucking in the bedding. The action of leaning across to draw blankets up near the pillows is also taxing if this reach is supported by a typically soft abdomen. In this position, the poor back acts like a derrick. It is a classic way of straining your back.

The best way to make a bed is to crouch beside it on your haunches, not on your knees, because you can make better use of the leverage of your strong thigh muscles to make the activity more dynamic. Keep the tummy braced and don't hurry. This is also a good position for cleaning the bath.

All housework is taxing. The best way of minimising strain is to punctuate it with energetic bursts of stretching movements, particularly extension, that lovely back-arching action which is the antidote to stooping. When you feel tired and achy, drop everything and fling yourself back, with both arms stretched out above your head. Do it several times. It works wonders!

WHY IS MY BACKACHE WORSE BEFORE MY MENSTRUAL PERIOD?

The alteration in hormonal balance before a monthly period results in fluid retention. Women often complain of feeling uncomfortable and bloated. The excess fluid collects in the soft tissues and the joints do not escape this. And any joint that is already swollen and painful will automatically become more so. The worst times are the few days immediately preceding the period but, in some women, it can gradually increase from the middle of the cycle up until the day or so before bleeding starts. This accounts for backache frequently worsening during the second part of the monthly cycle.

10 A Daily Self-Treatment Plan

Knees-to-Chest

This exercise can be done every day before you get out of bed or as the first step in an end-of-day regime:

1. Lie flat on the back, bring one knee to the chest and bounce it there.
2. Then, bring the other knee up and bounce both knees on the chest, with the fingers loosely interlaced around the knees and the head resting on the floor. Don't tug at the knees. The movement should be a gentle, relaxing, oscillatory bounce. You may have to hold each knee separately if you have a large tummy or if your hips are stiff, in which case it may help to cross the ankles and let the knees flop apart.
3. Continue this movement for one minute, paying attention to how the pulling sensation in the lower back slowly eases.

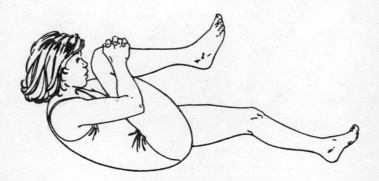

Figure 10.1.1 Gently pull one knee to the chest and bounce it there.

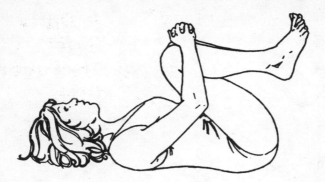

Figure 10.1.2 Repeat with both knees.

Lumbar Rolling

1. Lie on your back on the floor and bring your knees to your chest, holding them with your hands cupped. Your spine should adopt the shape of a wide *U*, which requires substantial strength in your neck and tummy muscles.
2. In this position, roll gently back and forth along your spine, trying to loosen the stiff links while keeping the movement smooth and rhythmic. (At first, this action will not feel smooth. It will probably feel more like rolling over a square wheel, but keep relaxed and you will adjust.)
3. Continue this movement for one minute, rest and then repeat it for another

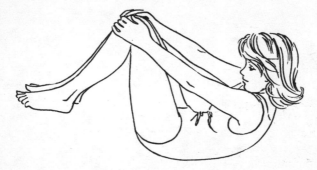

Figure 10.2 Lumbar rolling (pivoting).

minute. Don't course up and down the entire length of your spine. You must keep centred on the lower segments, or the ones that hurt, as you pivot on them.

Squatting

1. Holding the edge of the bathtub or some fixed support that can take your weight as you lean back.
2. With the feet together and parallel and the heels flat on the floor, lower your bottom to the floor in a deep squat.
3. Spread your knees wide with the arms outstretched between them.
4. Bounce your bottom towards the floor and, at the same time, lower your head between your knees. Feel your spine stretch and grow as your bottom drops down.
5. Do this for several bounces, then stand up, pulling your tummy in hard as you rise from the floor. Repeat this three times.

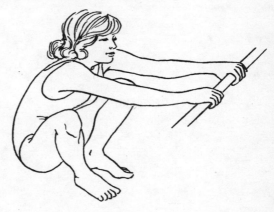

Figure 10.3 Squatting.

The Floor Twist

1. Take a position on the floor with lots of space around you because this exercise requires room.
2. Lie on your back with your arms out-stretched, at shoulder level, palms down.
3. Bring both knees up, high onto the chest.
4. Roll them over to the right and rest the knees on the floor. (As the legs go over, try to avoid letting your left hand and arm lift off the floor. You will feel a strong pull across the front of the shoulder and chest wall.)
5. Straighten the left leg at the knee and take hold of the left foot or ankle with your right hand. This will increase the stretch over the upper chest wall and shoulder and also in the back of the left thigh.
6. Hold the foot there and relax, breathing deeply as you feel the chest and leg letting go.

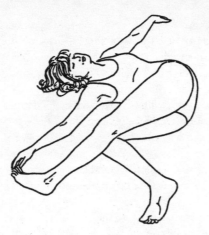

Figure 10.4 Floor twist.

7. Repeat this twice on each side, holding the stretch for at least 30 seconds. If your problem is unilateral (one-sided), repeat it three times to the bad side to one to the good. At first, you may be unable to straighten your stretching leg at the knee but this will come in time.

The Ma Roller

1. Lie on your back on the floor with your knees bent.
2. Lift your bottom and position yourself on the roller with the two wooden humps either side of the knobs running down the centre of your spine.
3. Move back and forth over the roller, a small section at a time, focusing on the sore spots.

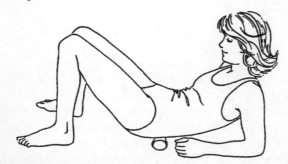

Figure 10.5 Ma roller under lumbar spine.

4. Continue this for at least 30 seconds and rest. Repeat once. If your problem is unilateral, you may find the pressure of the roller more piercing if you lie with the handle under the facet joint on one side of the spine only.

The BackBlock

If you are very stiff you can use the BackBlock on its flattest side (7 cm) at first, but most people start with it on its middle edge (12 cm).

1. Lie on your back on the floor, knees bent.
2. Lift your bottom and slide the BackBlock under the sacrum, the hard, flat bone at the base of the spine. Never place it higher, under your spine.
3. Lower your bottom onto the Block; then lower one leg down, by sliding the heel out along the floor, followed by the other. Your body is then flopped, draped backwards over the BackBlock.
4. Try to relax in this position for 60 seconds. You will feel a stretch at the front of the hips and a strong pull at the base of the spine.
5. To remove the BackBlock, bend one leg, then the other, and lift the bottom clear. There may often be a jab of pain at this point, so take care and lift your bottom slowly.
6. Lower your bottom back to the floor and keep the knees bent.
7. Take one knee to the chest and bounce it there gently.
8. Bring the other knee to the chest and bounce them both together. Your fingers should be interlaced around the knees with your head resting on the floor. Don't tug at your knees but make the movement as gentle and relaxed as possible. It should subtly hinge open the back of your spine.
9. Continue for one minute, noticing that the pulling sensation in the lower back is gradually easing.
10. Next, the sit-ups: lie on the floor with the knees bent, both feet secured under a bed or some other fixed support.
11. Bring the chin to the chest and curl up to the sitting position. If this is difficult, you may pull on the back of your thighs to get up; then return to the floor unaided.
12. As you progress, continue past the sitting position by opening your knees wide apart, stretching your hands through the knees as far forward as you can, even pulling on your ankles with your hands.
13. Return to the floor by pulling the tummy in and tipping the pelvis back so the humped low back presses into the floor and your spine slowly unfolds along the floor, like a carpet being unrolled.
14. Rest your head on the floor before repeating the sit-ups at least ten times.

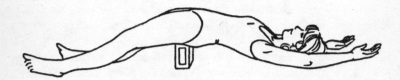

Figure 10.6 BackBlock (middle edge).

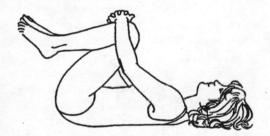

Figure 10.7 Knee bounces, until any discomfort in the low back has eased.

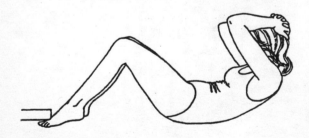

Figure 10.8 Sit-ups may have to be done initially with the arms stretched forward, head between the knees, hands grasping the ankles.

These fourteen steps represent one complete cycle of the BackBlock. The entire cycle – BackBlock, knee bounces and sit-ups – should be repeated another two or three times.

The Toe Touches

1. Stand with your feet 10 cm apart on the floor.
2. Pull your tummy in hard, tip forward at the waist and bend over towards the floor.
3. When you are hanging down freely, with your head and arms dangling, gently bounce while keeping the tummy sucked in. As you pull in the tummy, you will feel an extra release in the lower back. (If you are wary of bending over, place your hands on your thighs for support as you go down. When you feel secure, hang in that position.)
4. After a few bounces, return to vertical by pulling in your tummy hard and rolling your pelvis back. Tuck your bottom under and unfurl the spine to the upright position, head up last.
5. Repeat three to four times.

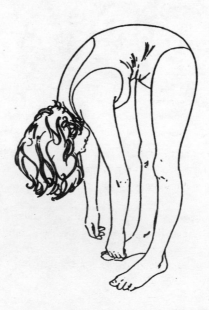

Figure 10.9 The toe touches

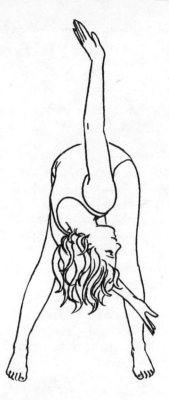

Figure 10.10 The diagonal toe touches

The Diagonal Toe Touches

1. Stand with your feet 60 cm apart.
2. With a sweeping, controlled movement, and nipping in your waist as you go, take your right hand down to the floor, pointing it well beyond the left ankle.
3. Pushing past, bounce several times, feeling the twist in the low back.
4. Return to vertical by unfurling and untwisting your spine upright as you suck in your tummy.
5. Repeat with your left hand pushing past your right ankle.
6. Do this three times to each side.

These eight exercises complete the daily self-treatment plan.

11 Back With Optimism

So, there you are! The complete concept of joint management. This should help you to take care of your hurting back. I trust I have imbued you with some degree of hope and optimism.

Of course, there will always be backs that are beyond the type of help that we manual therapists can provide. However, I am more concerned with those at the other end of the spectrum, those who have a totally manageable spinal problem but are completely unaware of such simple, effective measures so close at hand.

One last thing. The manual mobilisation of joints, not just of spinal joints, is carried out by a relatively small band of therapists worldwide. Being few in number, they are also hard to find. However, every central institute of physiotherapy, in whichever country you are, has a register of manual therapists who are trained in this area. (Having said that, my name does not appear on any of these lists and probably never will, but it is a good place to start.) Your doctor should be able to tell you, but, failing that, look in your telephone directory under the 'physiotherapists' section, ring around various practices and ask!

BackBlock and Ma Roller

The BackBlock (£30 inclusive of p&p) and Ma Roller (£20 inclusive p&p) used in this book can be purchased direct by sending cheque or money order (made payable to Sunsar Blocks Ltd) to:

Sunsar Blocks
Blenheim Estate Office
WOODSTOCK
Oxon OXA 1PS
UK

Both come with comprehensive instructions on how they should be used.